Christa Gebhardt, Jürgen Hansel

Whole again

Whole Again
The Homeopathic Way of Healing
13 Amazing Stories

Christa Gebhardt, Jürgen Hansel

Title of German Edition: Glücksfälle?
© 2006 Wilhelm Goldmann Verlag, München

English Edition
© 2008 Narayana Verlag GmbH, Blumenplatz 2, 79400 Kandern, Germany,
Phone +49 7626 9749700; info@narayana-publishers.eu; www. narayana-publishers.eu

ISBN 978-3-939931-59-1

Translated by Jennifer Buhl and Sue Elwen
Edited by to Gill Zukovskis

Cover photo: Lisa Bössen

All rights reserved. No part of this book may be reproduced by any mechanical, photographic, or electronic process, or in the form of a phonographic recording, nor may it be stored in any retrieval system, transmitted, or otherwise be copied for private or public use without the written permission of the publisher.

Christa Gebhardt, Jürgen Hansel

Whole again

The Homeopathic Way of Healing
13 Amazing Stories

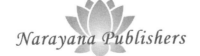

Contents

Introduction	1
1. A Stranger in Her Own Skin	10
2. Blessed art thou, Maria!	28
3. The End of the Line	48
4. Lovesick	61
5. The Land Beyond the Desert	72
6. Red and Blue	88
7. The Lost Warrior	104
8. A Law Unto Himself	123
9. Savita's Smile	139
10. A Part of the Family	152
11. The Poison of Fear	168
12. The Prince in the Caul or The Child of Fortune	181
13. If the Ice Breaks…	193
Glossary	206
Periodic Table of the Elements	212
Bibliography	213

Introduction

> *Everything is possible in this universe,*
> *provided enough is irrational.*
>   Niels Bohr

Everything began more than twenty years ago with a little finger. It happened during my daily rounds as a staff physician in the Hospital for Natural Healing in Munich. A female patient had suffered a severe stroke with subsequent paralysis of half of her body. Six weeks of intensive physical therapy in a renowned rehabilitation clinic had not brought any progress. Homeopathic treatment was her last hope. Back then I couldn't share this hope.

Still relatively new to homeopathy, I found it hard to believe that the small globules of endlessly diluted substances could have any effect on such a severe clinical picture. Nevertheless I had prescribed a homeopathic remedy for her in accordance with the Law of Similars, based on her particular symptoms. Now, one day after the dose of a high potency of the remedy *Nux vomica*, she gave me a contented smile: "Look here, Doctor." She was moving the little finger of her paralyzed hand.

That little finger hasn't let go of me since. My scientific-medical picture of the world was permanently shattered by it. How was it possible that a plant extract diluted past the limit of detection could trigger such a reaction? And, moreover, in a case for which even the modern pharmaceutical industry held no cure. I still can't answer this question today. As yet there is no conclusive scientific explanation for the astonishing effects of homeopathy. The reawakening of the little finger and then of the entire paralyzed half of the body, which soon followed, was the beginning of an adventure for me. Through this experience, I learned as a young doctor to marvel at the miracles of homeopathy, and I haven't stopped marvelling to this day. After many years in my own practice and as the organizer of training seminars in homeopathy, I have felt a growing desire to tell people about at least some of these amazing things and thereby perhaps infect others with my enthusiasm.

My wife also shared this enthusiasm. When I met her, she was a dedicated journalist following all of the paths and channels offered by her chosen profession to pursue her great passion: people. What they think, what they say, how they feel and why they do what they do. She soon became interested in homeopathy, for it was clear to her that both of us are seeking something very similar in our very different professions: an understanding of the inner, sometimes hidden stories of people, their unique view of the world, their very own truths and behavior patterns. In the seminars she attended whenever her work schedule allowed, she learned through homeopathic case studies about the different methods and the subtleties of this art of leading a person so close to himself through sensitive questioning that the center of his suffering comes to light and can be translated into a homeopathic remedy prescription. Amazing and sometimes even breathtaking for her was the extent of the transformation that patients can undergo after a particularly successful prescription. She knows that this is not an everyday occurrence in homeopathy and that such cases often take years and some unsuccessful prescriptions before they finally make such satisfactory progress. Nevertheless, she felt that if something like this is at all possible, even if only seldom, then people need to know about it. Definitely! Not just homeopaths.

Thus evolved the idea of putting our experiences together, writing true stories of "strokes of luck" like these and describing the method which can sometimes give luck a helping hand.

It took another few years until our partnership bore fruit in a form which in retrospect seems completely logical - this book, in which two circles touch at one point and connect harmoniously. At the beginning, however, there were challenging experiences which took a lot of courage to deal with. For a doctor of medicine, for whom science has become the measure of all things over the course of years of study, it is not so easy to deal with phenomena that contradict the basic assumptions he has learned. That our readers too might face such challenging experiences is our declared intention. They should be surprised, and it is all right if the world view of some is shaken a bit. Many similar stories have come along since that patient moved her little finger so surprisingly and was finally able to walk out of the hospital on her own, and they have continued to call into question my previous medical concepts.

One of the first patients in my own practice was a particularly challenging case. Six weeks after the young man had received a very high potency, 10 M or C 10,000 of *Sepia*, the ink of the cuttlefish, for a chronic infection of the prostate, he reported astonishing changes in his life: he had broken off his unhappy relationship, looked for a new apartment, quit his job and gone into business for himself. A sensation of congestion and blockage, which he had felt for years, was suddenly gone and he had a completely new outlook on life. He mentioned only in passing that his physical complaints had completely disappeared.

A healing reaction like this was unknown to me from my studies and my previous medical experience. Perhaps something like this happens after years of psychoanalysis. But six weeks after a dose of three tiny globules? That sounds like magic. Or coincidence. After all, it is possible that it all would have happened without the *Sepia* globules. When similar reactions occur in totally different people, however, one notices that it is more than just a coincidence. The patients describe the special effect of homeopathy on their entire being in different words: "As if I had come home," is a typical phrase, "I feel totally different," or "I have never been so calm and balanced." And from friends and acquaintances, they hear, "You have become a different person." In the process of sickness and healing, they have left something behind and taken a new step, a step further toward themselves. They have also achieved a degree of freedom that they never knew before or that they had lost. This "quantum leap" to a new level of their being sometimes comes so suddenly and unexpectedly that it is seen as a miracle.

In such experiences, we recognize a dimension of healing that does not exist in conventional medicine. It is that which is truly exceptional about homeopathy, which is not about repairing a defect, eliminating a local malady or fighting a pathogen. It is about the whole, about triggering a reaction of the self-healing forces of the organism on all levels. Only when the prevailing mood of a person, his vitality and his outlook on life change for the better, when he feels more balanced overall, are we satisfied with the effect of a homeopathic remedy. The cure of the physical illness is then virtually a side-effect of the main effect on the vital force of a person. The criteria for such an ideal development – feelings, mood, energy – seem rather vague, however, and extremely subjective. They can hardly be standardized, statistically recorded or even objectified.

If one wants to evaluate the effect of homeopathy with the instruments of scientific research, with statistics and double-blind studies, there is an even greater problem. The method developed by Samuel Hahnemann over 200 years ago still demands today that a remedy be chosen which matches the individual symptoms of the patient in every case. More important than the clinical diagnosis are – according to Hahnemann – "the strange, rare and peculiar signs and symptoms" of a patient, his characteristic subjective suffering, his personal individuality. The treatment thus orients itself more strongly towards the person than towards the disease. And therefore it is entirely possible that ten people with the same disease diagnosis can receive ten different homeopathic remedies. Studies which evaluate the effect of Medication A on Disease B cannot do justice to the homeopathic method.

While scientific-medical research consistently tries to extrapolate from the individual in order to make generally valid, objective statements, homeopathy proceeds in the opposite direction. Here the focus of attention is directed toward the individual as an incomparably unique being. The key to successful homeopathic treatment lies in the personal story of each patient. The case history therefore ranks above statistics in importance in homeopathy; this experiential approach to medicine can best be understood and explained through the portrayal of individual cases. It is not enough here to report on a case of rheumatism or tuberculosis in the style of classical medical reports with the typical symptoms. It is also not enough to record data and facts from the patient's life. In normal medical case histories, the subjective world of the patient with his survival strategies and behavior patterns, with his sensitivity and his special way of reacting to stress and illness is missing. To reach this level of the inner workings of a human being, we must expand the case history into a life story, the portrait of a totally unique person.

That is the basic idea behind this book. We want to make the individual approach of homeopathy and its special way of working apparent through very personal life stories. In the center of every story is the fate of a person, the development of physical and emotional suffering in the context of his biography and the process of transformation which is initiated through his encounter with the homeopathic remedy. Just as we were touched, moved and shattered by the outer and inner lives of each person as we worked on this book, we want to pass our experience on – in a way that reaches the heart as well as the mind, similar to the holistic effect of a well-selected remedy on the spirit and mind. This is why the form and language of the short stories reflect the personality of the main figures and their special way of expressing themselves. How a person speaks, how he or she moves, the overall impression he or she makes on us are important criteria for a homeopathic prescription. The unusual form of this book, the combination of literary narrative and expert commentary, is a synthesis of both of our professional backgrounds as a journalist and writer on the one side and as a homeopathic physician on the other.

The biographies that we portray may seem unusual and often dramatic. In medical practice, such circumstances are certainly not the exception. Many people have had similar experiences and many will recognize their own experiences and problems in the narratives.

What is special and what all of the stories have in common is "a real and extraordinary event," as in a novel. Fate takes a completely unexpected turn, a knot comes untied, psychologically or physically, sometimes decades after an unresolved trauma. A meningioma disappears, burned skin regains sensation, a new outlook on life develops. One cannot simply prescribe such quantum leaps. A person must be ready for them and the time must be right. Even when experienced homeopaths witness this wonderful phenomenon of deep healing again and again, it is not a daily occurrence even for the best of them, but rather the highest ideal of this medicine. It often takes years – in our examples as well – for a remedy to be found that can turn someone's life around.

Usually the transformation does not take place suddenly and abruptly like a quantum leap. It develops more often in a continuous healing process, which must be followed attentively and consistently. Of course we would be happiest if all of our suffering could be extinguished with a few globules. In acute illnesses this is entirely possible. But for deeply rooted personal problems and the illnesses connected with them, miracles take a bit longer. With adequate homeopathic stimulation, movement is introduced where there is a fixed pattern, a rigid posture. As if the organism has simultaneously received more energy and a new idea and can now deal with its old problems with new vigor. Often the entire system first enters a state of upheaval. Physical symptoms can become worse and sometimes the scarred soul also suffers in this watershed phase. When a new balance on a higher level of health has gradually established itself after such a crisis, it does not mean that one is automatically protected from future illness. Our self-healing powers in this new state can, however, cope much better with external and internal stresses.

Homeopathic treatment, just like the healing process, follows certain principles. Nevertheless, no case is like another. This inevitably results from the method, which – as previously mentioned – emphasizes the individual characteristics of the disease and the patient. We must therefore warn against transferring symptoms and problems from the case stories in this book directly to a personal situation and taking the same homeopathic remedy because of similarities to a certain story or even because of the same diagnosis. The flood of guidebooks on the homeopathic book market suggests that one can treat oneself with globules very well. This may be the case for certain standard situations or minor illnesses, but not for chronic conditions and severe pathologies. In such cases, even a trained homeopath would not treat himself, because he does not have the necessary distance to view his reaction pattern objectively.

The peculiarity of each individual case history is not only determined by the patient and his disease, but also by the personality of the therapist. The doctor-patient relationship, a central element of every treatment, plays a special role in homeopathy. Without a stable, trusting relationship, a patient is highly unlikely to reveal the deeply personal pains of his inner experience which so often give decisive indications to the optimal remedy. Every homeopath proceeds here somewhat differently and develops his own working method. It was therefore important for us to add the patients of several colleagues from different countries to our own case histories in this collection in order to present a broad spectrum of methods. The homeopathic repertoire has been expanded in the last 20 years to include many more remedies, and also new methods of approach. Two especially renowned protagonists of these developments, Rajan Sankaran from Bombay and Jan Scholten from Utrecht, have contributed case histories from their practices to this book.

The contact with Dr. Sankaran and his colleagues at the Bombay School of Homeopaths enabled us to speak with several patients in India and to add their stories to our book. We had a special reason for the long journey: homeopathy is more strongly integrated in the health system in India than it is in Europe. Since it was given equal status with other forms of medicine in 1973, it has received unrestricted government support. In this country, more homeopaths practise than in any other country in the world and they also frequently treat severe organic disturbances. The potential of Hahnemann's form of medicine can thus best be studied today in India.

In Bombay as in Holland, Austria and Germany, patients, their parents and their partners have met us with trust and great openness and have told us in detail about their lives, their suffering and their healing process. They have taken a great deal of their time to do so, because they want to express their thanks in this way for their healing and help other people learn more about the amazing possibilities of homeopathy. For many of them it was not easy to recount painful experiences or to read their own story of suffering later as a narrative. From some we have heard that this encounter with the shadows of the past has brought them a bit farther along on their journey to themselves. Their willingness to become involved in this venture deserves great respect and we thank them all sincerely for this. Their contribution is the soul of this book.

The spirit of this book radiates from the therapists who have treated these people so successfully. We were very fortunate to be connected with these colleagues through years of seminar activities together. They also gave us a great deal of trust and time, established contact with their patients for us, gave us insights into their work and examined the results of our work. And they entertained us often and looked after us in foreign surroundings. For this we thank our friends and colleagues Divya Chhabra, Sujit Chatterjee, Jutta Gnaiger-Rathmanner, Rajan Sankaran, Anne Schadde, Jan Scholten, Jayesh Shah, Annette Sneevliet, Rienk Stuut, Franz Swoboda and Ulrich Welte. After consulting with the patients, we have given the names of the homeopaths in some stories, while in others we have not. To ensure the anonymity of the main people in the stories, their names were changed, as were their places of residence and their professions. In the three cases from my practice, we have also covered our tracks, since here a patient would be especially easy to identify. Should one reader or another still recognize a story, we ask that he preserve the anonymity of the people involved.

We also thank friends and colleagues who helped to make a book out of our texts. We thank the translator Jochen Lehner and his actress wife Gabriele, the author and editor Stephan Schumacher, the editors from Süddeutsche Zeitung Cathrin Kahlweit and Stephanie Schwaderer, the homeopathic pediatrician Dr. Andreas Richter, the Sinologist and TCM expert Prof. Stephan Pàlos and our daughter Johanna. They advised us well, encouraged us, read the manuscript critically and gave us valuable suggestions. Thanks are also due to Jennifer Buhl and Sue Elwen for their outstanding English translation, to Gill Zukovskis for doing an excellent job as editor and to the publishers Katrin and Herbert Sigwart, as well as Ulrich Welte, who have paved the way for our book to reach a wider audience with this translated version.

It was our goal to write a book about people and their lives in which one could learn in passing about various aspects of the homeopathic method and its special holistic effect. Readers with a homeopathic background will surely encounter unusual remedies and perhaps new approaches to case analysis. The commentaries should, however, also be understandable for lay readers and reveal to them from one chapter to the next the secrets of homeopathy. We have defined basic terms of this medicine in a glossary at the end of the book and recommend that those who are not familiar with the method read these short explanations in advance.

Munich, October 2008

Christa Gebhardt   *Jürgen Hansel*

1. A Stranger in her own Skin

> *To prepare the animal charcoal, lay a thick piece of ox-leather between the red-hot coals and allow it to burn, until the last little flame disappears and then quickly place the glowing piece between two flat stones, so that it may be suddenly extinguished, as else it would continue to glimmer in the open air, destroying the coal for the most part.*
>
> Samuel Hahnemann
> (from *The Chronic Diseases*)

The whole child stood in flames. Eloise was burning like a torch. Before everyone's eyes. They smelled the burning odor of Ellie's blazing hair and her glowing skin. They saw her flailing. They saw the look of sheer terror in her eyes. And they saw how her flesh fed the flames, how she was consumed by the fire. Frightfully fast. Time was going by. And Ellie was burning. She was burning in the living room of her own home in the middle of her large family like a witch at the stake. Before they finally extinguished the flames burning the twelve-year-old girl, they had brought her out in front of the house to keep the fire from spreading to the furniture.

The long white perlon dress with the petticoat and the pink ribbons, which had caught fire on a radiant heater, stuck to young

Ellie like glowing liquid rubber, dug into her skin and flesh, right down to the bones. She screamed like a madwoman, until she went into shock and lost consciousness.

Months later, when she returned to her home, disfigured by scars, the fire was extinguished from her memory. It remained forgotten for almost 30 years. Ellie could not remember anything: the burning, the pain, the first weeks in the hospital. No one spoke of the incident in her family. Not one of her six siblings said a word about it over the years, nor did her father and mother or her many distant aunts and uncles. Perhaps Amma, her grandmother, would have talked to her about it. But Amma was dead. She died when Ellie was in the clinic.

In the first weeks after the accident, the doctors loosened from her tortured body burned pieces of tissue and scabs layer by layer, in numerous smaller and larger operations. Dead skin was cut off, the remaining, only half-destroyed skin was cared for and nourished as well as possible. With strong pain medications, the girl was kept in an artificial coma. After weeks, Ellie was still in shock. She was transferred to the women's ward because the danger of infection there was not as great as in the children's clinic. Finally, when her condition became more critical, she was put in quarantine in the isolation ward, for her wounded body reacted very sensitively to bacterial infections. When she woke up, no one was there with her. Sometimes a nurse briefly held her hand. It was a miracle that she survived.

The long months of very slow recovery in the clinic after the first weeks of hovering between life and death remained only vague in Ellie's memory, like a black-and-white film from another life, with another leading actress. Ellie was no longer Ellie. This was a feeling which accompanied her almost her entire life and which must have existed back then - that much she knows. It was something that felt like terrible homesickness. When her parents and family came to visit her some Sundays and sat in her hospital room, they were silent most of the time and somehow Ellie was happy when they finally left again. No, it wasn't her father and mother she yearned for. It was a feeling that she didn't completely understand, similar perhaps to homesickness for a place where she could be intact. A yearning for life.

Ellie was branded like an animal. She guessed it without really knowing, without any real idea of her situation. Later she remembered how people she didn't know stood around her bed and stared at her. This picture remained in her head. As long as she was in the clinic, she herself never saw or felt her burned skin and the scars. Her hands were thickly bandaged as well. The nurses who dressed her wounds sometimes gave each other looks which she could not yet interpret. This girl would be marked for her entire life. Ellie's body was quickly wrapped again in cloths and bandages. They had to protect the patient from germs. During the day, Ellie hardly spoke. At night she was tortured by nightmares, but she didn't dare to ring for help. The nurses heard Ellie screaming in her sleep and often had to change the sheets because her bed was wet. In the 1960's, no one had thought yet of the necessity of psychological treatment. Her emotional suffering could not be overlooked, however.

After three months in the clinic, the doctors urgently recommended that the parents take their severely traumatized child home and nurse her back to health. But after just a few days it became clear that Ellie's mother was not willing to take this on. The other children, four older and two younger, took priority. Ellie could not walk, could hardly move and her wounds had to be bandaged regularly. Moreover, she would have needed a great deal of emotional attention. But there were the six other brothers and sisters. She was thus given to a distant aunt to be cared for. There she heard for the first time about the death of her grandmother. Ellie's grandmother was the only person in her life who had really loved her. She could always flee to her when she was beaten at home, and she would love to have stayed for good with her Amma. Amma was like a mother to her, who loves and accepts her child, embraces her and gently strokes her hair. Amma was the only person whose touch felt good. Ellie had stayed alone for long periods of time at her grandmother's time and again, while the other siblings stayed at home with the parents. But now Amma was gone forever.

It was clear that it was Ellie's own fault that she was in this state and was covered with ugly scars on her arms, legs, chest and upper back: she was a terrible child. The mother and the older sisters had always said that she was evil and that she constantly made her mother suffer so. How often had she been locked in the cellar as punishment and had to eat there. And now she heard her father say when he saw the scars, "That is God's punishment!" It served her right. Surely everyone thought the same. She had to go and do that to her mother. She had to be so clumsy and stupid as to burn herself on the heater. In front of everyone. They probably all kept silent about it to spare her the shame of her misdeed. Amma alone might have been able to offer a small comfort by saying that maybe it wasn't all the way it seemed. At least she would have taken Ellie in her arms. And when she thought of her Amma, whom she sorely missed, Ellie cried for the first time since she was burned, in the room of her distant aunt. Very quietly, with her face turned to the wall, so the aunt would not hear anything.

Just as the incident remained a taboo subject, the family also said nothing about Ellie's scars. They all simply gaped at her when she returned home. When the big tub was filled with bath water for all of the siblings once a week, her brothers and sisters stood around and stared wide-eyed at Ellie's body. Their looks were like magnifying glasses which burned holes in her skin. She slipped into the tub with the steaming water as fast as she could. She didn't feel how hot the water was. She didn't recoil. It didn't feel good and it didn't feel bad. It didn't feel like anything. A large portion of the nerves in her skin seemed to be dead. It didn't hurt. Can it be that whoever doesn't feel pain, doesn't feel at all? Ellie still felt, but she didn't know it. She felt only fear. She was terribly afraid for the whole week of being exposed to those mute stares again.

After her open wounds had healed, Ellie had to learn many things again like a small child. Her legs regained their function after a while so that she was able to walk. Her arms and elbows often remained immobile or numb and sometimes hung from her like foreign objects. She didn't think anything of it because she couldn't remember how agile and lively she had been before. Helpless, without a secure feeling, her body remained handicapped. And her soul as well. Ellie shut herself off and didn't let anyone get close to her. She could not stand having her scarred skin touched. Her strongest feeling was the fear of being stared at, like in the hospital or at home in the bath. Because she didn't want to undress in front of others, she skipped physical education. She didn't like to go out and be with other people, certainly not to parties. The laughter made her suspicious, for she found most of the jokes were not funny, but dirty and mean.

Thus she didn't laugh and she also didn't cry. Ellie had become totally blunted. She did what she was told and didn't ask questions. Even when it was torture, like the swimming that she had to do to restore the mobility of her body, so the flesh would become softer again. The lifeguard, who did not sense the fears of the girl, forced her again and again into the deep water, where she couldn't stand and couldn't see the bottom. Since then she had had a terrible fear of water, even as an adult. Then it became even worse. She felt that the water was calling her and commanding her to kill herself. Once, much later, when she was standing on the shore of a lake with her two sons, the pull of the water was so great that she never went to lakes or rivers again after that. Certainly never to the sea, for there her suicidal urge became overpowering and even stronger than her feeling of responsibility toward her two children, whom she loved above all else.

Ellie took the first man who came along. He was a tyrant and treated her like a slave. That wasn't new to her. At home with her parents she had had to take on most of the housework. While the other children did homework or went outside to play, Ellie had to peel potatoes, iron clothes, scrub the floors. Ellie's father allowed her mother to treat this one child like a maid. He himself had little time for the family. His life was dedicated to God. He devoted his strength and his time to the church and what it demanded of him. For those around him there was not much left. He didn't really notice Ellie until his wife had been dead for some time. Yet he didn't love her any less than the other children – in contrast to his wife. She had rejected Ellie, the fifth child, from the beginning. After the birth, she refused to nurse the baby. The infant had to be given to a relative to be cared for. He told her all of this later. But he didn't tell Ellie why her mother had rejected her.

Ellie was 22 when she married Rob in order to escape her life of slavery under her mother. Before the wedding she had already left him several times because he had insulted and beaten her. But she softened time and again when he fell on his knees before her and swore in tears that he would change. He needed her so much. And he abused her. In the marriage with Rob, Ellie fell into her old role again. As Cinderella, just like back home. And Rob was not the prince who freed her. He screamed at her whenever he felt like it, forbade her to go out on the street with the children, ignored her pleas to be careful with her scarred skin – instead he threatened her and was violent toward her in bed. She endured it. No pain, no feelings, no life.

Ellie knew only one way to bear all of this. She withdrew more and more, avoided contact with the world and with people, took as little notice of everything as possible. She lived as though she were in a dark tunnel, which isolated her from life outside. Yet she functioned perfectly. Tirelessly she kept going, always one step after the other. She had been caring and loving toward her two younger siblings, to whom she was very attached. Taking care of the two little ones had kept her alive during her youth. She now cared for her two sons just as devotedly, as they meant everything to her. Ellie was not burned inside. She had felt the two babies growing inside of her and the pain of the births brought back some life to her. After that she lived through her children. Everything that concerned the boys touched her soul. Her life was there, with her children. She loved her sons like all mothers love their children and then a bit more, with a last existential power of survival.

When she took care of others like this, Ellie could begin to sense her energy. She could handle children, and also sick people, very well. She therefore volunteered to help at school and later as an aide in the hospital. Rob tacitly put up with her volunteer activities, although he had forbidden her to work outside of the house. But only on the condition that the housework was done on time, properly and to his full satisfaction. The same held true for her other duties as a wife. At the school, Ellie got to know a social worker. He was nice to her, talked with her about the problems of the children they were entrusted with, and after a while a friendly relationship developed between the two. He had noticed for a long time that Ellie hid her scars, and one day he spoke to her about them. Not out of curiosity, but because he wanted to help. He couldn't know what this would trigger.

It was a shock for Ellie. She broke down. Up until now, no one had touched on the taboo which lay upon her burns. The nervous breakdown of this woman who seemed so strong and easygoing was a puzzle for the clinic physicians. A psychologist tried to help Ellie through hypnotic treatment and slowly, in fragments, the horror that she had suffered as a twelve-year-old girl resurfaced from her subconscious. Ellie felt alone in the flames again, close to death, abandoned with her pain, thrown out of the house so she wouldn't burn anything else besides herself. Ellie cried and cried when she discovered the burning child inside of her. It exhausted all of her strength.

Ellie became sick. She suffered severe stomach bleeding. After every warm meal she felt nauseous. Sometimes she vomited a mixture of old and fresh blood. Her stool was often bloody and jet black. Just the smell of meat cooking made her retch and soon she could eat only ladyfingers (sponge cookies). She saw the hypnosis treatments through for two years, as they helped her to reach back to her memories. But physically she continued to worsen. Finally she was sent to a doctor who was to try homeopathy.

When Ellie met Dr. Stuut, she was almost forty. In his case taking he recorded her complaints and symptoms, asked about her childhood and finally touched on the burning incident. It was difficult for her to talk about it and she said only what was necessary. She reported only little about her mother, of the beatings and her feelings of guilt for being a terrible child without knowing what she had done wrong. Only upon direct questioning did she tell about her fear of crowds, her thoughts of suicide and her fear of water. It was easier for her to talk about physical complaints. There were the throat infections she had as a teenager, several abscesses, an operation on an ovarian cyst, the heavy, strong-smelling underarm perspiration, the hard swelling of the mammary glands before her periods. Since a fall on the stairs, her backbone hurt now and again and the pain extended down her leg. Because she could not stand bright light, she always wore sunglasses.

With the homeopathic treatment, Ellie's complaints diminished and she slowly came to trust her physician. He could see from the flowers she sent him for his birthday and the postcards she sent from her vacations how devoted and attentive she was becoming. But years passed before she could talk about feelings. She made progress during this time, even took a paid job in the psychiatric clinic and was pleased about how the patients liked her. She seemed less closed. Nevertheless the stomach problems kept coming back. After five years of treatment and about fifteen different homeopathic remedies, her body was not truly healthy. Not to mention her soul, the real Ellie.

It was like a puzzle that had to be put together out of remarks, episodes and Ellie's spontaneous reactions. There was her nervous smile when she talked about her worries and troubles, as if they were all very strange and funny. Or the story of the two co-workers who had planned to meet her in a restaurant, to help her come into contact with people. Without looking right or left, but staring straight at her two male friends, it took an almost insurmountable effort for her to walk as if through a narrow corridor through all of the strange people toward her colleagues. Even Ellie found her behavior somewhat peculiar when she told Dr. Stuut about it. But now he had a clear picture before him. He saw the dark tunnel through which Ellie walked in life.

Ellie's hidden emotional life became clearest in her dreams. Once she dreamed of being incurably ill. The more she fought against it, the worse it became. The disease was in her whole body. It was especially distressing for her that she could look down at herself from above in the dream. In a second dream, her grandmother lay on her deathbed. She was being laid out. Suddenly Amma rose and wanted to get out of bed. But she was forbidden to do so. Four men pushed her back. Ellie took her in her arms and she turned into a baby. They took the baby away from her because it was supposed to die. All of a sudden it was a sweet little animal which tried to jump on Ellie's mother's lap. But she displayed no reaction to the approach of the small creature. When Ellie told her doctor about this dream, she began to cry. For the first time she realized how strange she had felt in her own house, how much she missed the close relationship with her grandmother and how there had never been another person who had been there for her since then.

A third strange dream made everything even clearer. There was a big celebration at her house with her aunts and uncles. Everyone was eating and Ellie was supposed to stand up and speak in front of everyone. She was afraid to, but they dragged her into the middle of the room and wanted to force her. Ellie couldn't say a word. She was terribly afraid of not doing it right. When her mother began to berate her, she broke down. Her oldest brother told her it was because she had never been accepted in this family. He was truly astonished that Ellie had known this for a long time. She thought of her aunts and her Amma. They all knew it too. It was completely clear to her and still it was strange. Suddenly she began to talk gibberish and staggered like a drunkard. She fell to the floor and couldn't move anymore. It was strange for her to see herself lying there. Ellie wanted to get up, but her muscles didn't function anymore. She remained lying there like a wreck. Somehow her mother suddenly had a baby in her arms. She lay the child next to Ellie and that made Elllie react. Pressing the infant against her, she was able to get up. The warm head on her shoulder felt good. When her mother saw that it did her good, she said, "I will let her have the baby if only she becomes normal again." At the end Ellie saw herself walking away with the child.

The three dreams present a vivid picture of Ellie's emotional world, her fear of people, even of those who should have been closest to her; her shyness and inability to express herself and the feeling of being a wreck, emotionally broken and destroyed. She sees herself from above, everything is strange and peculiar: the world, herself, the others. It is still the same feeling she had back then in the clinic, when she was stared at as if she came from another planet. The homesickness that consumed her during that time takes on its own color and quality in the dreams. It is not her parents' house or familiar surroundings that Ellie is yearning for. It is the blissful state of a baby, intact, accepted, cared for by its Amma. The understanding of this special homesickness of an abandoned, shy child in strange surroundings led the physician to a homepathic remedy which has a very striking similarity to Ellie's horrible trauma. He gave her *Carbo animalis*, the charred skin of an ox, prepared and potentized according to the directions of Samuel Hahnemann.

The reaction was dramatic. Ellie developed a high fever shortly after taking the homeopathic animal charcoal and – as she had once had as a child – a large abscess between her buttocks. When everything was over after a week of high fever and heavy sweating and Eloise was able to get up, something totally unusual and surprising occurred: she stood in the shower and could suddenly feel the heat of the water. It was actually too hot for her skin and she had to make it colder. Now she could feel the cold stream on her chest just as keenly. She ran outside and felt for the first time since being burned in her childhood the warmth of the sun on her face, on her arms and legs, felt the warmth going through her dress and onto her whole body. How new, how good it felt. Out on the street, loud, liberating laughter broke out of her. She had discovered the sun again. From vacation she later wrote to her doctor, "I'm getting tan for the first time. That's never happened before!"

After a few weeks, Eloise fell into a severe depression. She felt cut off from the world, as if in a tunnel. And then it suddenly became clear to her: "This was and is the feeling that has been with me for 30 years of my life. I have lived as though I were in a dark tunnel." Her years of drudgery in her parents' house came to mind; she saw herself as a child. She knew now that this was in the past. There is another life. But the catharsis continued. An unexplained fever lasted for a week and finally landed Eloise in the hospital. The ultrasound examination showed a large abscess, this time in the intestines. The surgeon was hesitant about operating, gave her antibiotics and Eloise took "her" remedy *Carbo animalis* for the second time, in the same high potency. Some days later, to the surgeon's amazement, the enormous growth had disappeared without a trace.

And Eloise thought to herself, "Funny, I'm alive again." Feelings and sensations came back to her in completely normal little things and she discovered a totally new world: trees, birds, flowers. She saw them as if for the first time. For an entire week she gazed in wonder through the window at the hospital grounds. With binoculars she followed the birds' flights and couldn't get enough of it all. How beautiful they were, these flocks of birds. And the huge trees with their lush greenery. The carpets of flowers. It was such an energetic feeling: I am alive, and I am not alone. Life is all around me and there is so much of it. Someone is out on the street laying cobblestones, that's odd. Hey, there is someone laying cobblestones. He was there before, but she hadn't seen him with her tunnel vision. Strange.

Life grabbed hold of her and she grabbed hold of life. First she began to argue with a neighbor. Then she rebelled against her tyrannical husband. Again a dream came to her aid. She dreamed that she was rescued at the last minute from drowning. Drenched and completely exhausted, she dragged herself home and sank to the floor. Yet her husband commanded her to perform her housework immediately. In the dream, Eloise took a stick and smashed the chair he was sitting on. In reality she left her husband the very next day. She realized that she meant nothing to him. If all she had done for him meant nothing, she wanted to stop. Right away. Like a switch that is flipped. She went and left everything behind her, even her two children, the most wonderful things she had in the world. Their father forbade them to contact their mother. And Eloise suffered endlessly over this, but she held out. Even when Rob took her by force from her apartment and dragged her by the hair back to his house. She fled again and again.

Once again the painful abscesses on the buttocks returned. This was after Rob had tried to run over her. He came in his car in the dark. Her bicycle was totally destroyed, but Eloise survived. Now that she could feel herself again, she also had the strength to defend herself. She reported her husband to the police. She had to do it. Even if her soul had freed itself of him, he could still destroy her body. For a few months she didn't go to work because she was afraid of renewed attacks. Then he was convicted and sent to prison. Although Rob has been imprisoned four times since then, he has not given up stalking Eloise. He calls her at work every day and often sneaks past her apartment. Nevertheless, something is different: before she was afraid of him, but now he is afraid of her. And has respect for her. She enjoys frequent and gratifying contact with her sons. They are also no longer afraid of their father anymore.

Today Eloise feels healthy. All of her physical complaints are gone. The scars, which were once red and sensitive, are also fading. It is a long time since her trips were mainly an escape from her husband. She especially enjoys travelling south. Spain, India, Kenya. She enjoys it. Especially the warm light. Her life isn't easy though. Again and again she has to fight and assert herself. In a process which has been going on for about 10 years since the first dose of *Carbo animalis*. But she can do it. And slowly she is gathering courage to bring light into the darkness of her past.

On her initiative, she and her siblings have come into contact with each other. They wonder today why they have so many positive memories of their childhoods, but not Ellie. Her youngest brother is currently in therapy. It has become clear to him – he was seven at the time – that his parents tried to place the blame on him for Ellie's accident. Why didn't he go and get a blanket to smother the flames? Eloise loves this brother very much and embraces between them were always possible. Now she can also embrace others. The beginning of a new love relationship, the caresses of her boyfriend are like the time she first noticed the beauty of the trees: "Hey, that feels good!"

Some reservations remain, however. When Eloise talks about her family taboo, she shows signs of her nervous smile again. Until she was four, she was a happy, bright child. Until the abscesses appeared. Eloise now knows that her oldest brother tried back then to rape her. Her sisters watched. And afterward Ellie was beaten to a pulp by her mother. She still hasn't talked with anyone about it. The last secret has also never been revealed. The secret that Ellie's Amma, her aunts, her father and her mother shared with each other before they died. Why was Ellie the only unloved child? Why was she stigmatized by her mother and why were her burns the just punishment of God?

Perhaps Eloise will never ask these questions. Or perhaps she will need no more answers. She is now in the process of tapping into an energy that she feels deep within herself. Before, she could hardly touch other people. Now she has noticed that her hands possess great healing power. She uses them when she is asked. She is making her way, very carefully.

Commentary

Eloise had suffered an unbelievably hard fate with horrible injuries and her life was often sheer torture. However, this would not have been a reason for her to go to the homeopathic physician.

At the beginning of her homeopathic treatment stood a disease, as is often the case, with easily perceptible, clear physical symptoms, which she wanted to get rid of. In many cases, not just with Eloise, such visible complaints are merely the tip of the proverbial iceberg. Yet if her stomach hadn't bled, she probably wouldn't have gone to Dr. Stuut. She couldn't talk about feelings back then, but she could talk about her nausea and vomiting blood and also about previous diseases and complaints. This was the initial basis for treatment. The jet-black stool, the indigestibility of warm meals, the revulsion at food odors, the aversion towards meat, the extreme fatigue which came over her in conjunction with the nausea.

On the basis of such clear physical symptoms, the first remedies were prescribed according to the Law of Similars, remedies such as *Causticum* or *Sepia*, since the symptoms they caused in the remedy provings were similar to Ellie's. The remedies did have some effect. The acute complaints diminished and Eloise was able to take on a new job. She functioned again. But her stomach didn't let up. Time and again it brought her back into the homeopathic practice, until she had gotten to know the physician well and was slowly able to open up more over the years. During this process, the physical complaints finally moved into the background and Eloise's psychosocial problems came to the fore in the homeopathic consultation and treatment. It is therefore not surprising that Eloise was given about fifteen different remedies in five years. Here there were various reasons for the change from one remedy to another.

First of all, it is the nature of the Law of Similars that several remedies are possible for a given case. These should fulfill the condition of being able to cause a similar disease picture to the case, but not exactly the same picture. In contrast to sameness, similarity is not exactly defined. Thus there can be a whole set of people who are similar to you in one way or another: in their appearance, their stature or their character. Yet you will hardly find a double who is like you in every way, unless you have an identical twin. If you are looking for a double, you will need to consider what makes you what you are and which characteristics are most important. This is also how a homeopath proceeds when seeking a remedy to match the disease of a particular person. And then he will often find several remedies which meet the search criteria in some way.

With Eloise there was, however, another reason why so many remedies were needed. During the treatment process over the years, significant characteristics changed in the picture she presented to her physician, thereby changing the basis for applying the Law of Similars. This steady transformation was both a reflection of her developing relationship with her doctor and a direct result of the homeopathic treatment. The different remedies which were selected on the basis of the current symptom picture helped Eloise to overcome a portion of her complaints, step by step. It was as though a layer of the disease was removed and beneath it a new layer appeared which displayed a different picture and required a new remedy.

The Greek homeopath Georgos Vithoulkas, who received the Alternative Nobel Prize in 1996 for homeopathic medicine, writes about courses of treatment such as this: "Whoever really wants to heal his patients must not ignore these layers. If a patient has many of these layers, the cure will take a relatively long time. In this case the homeopath must systematically remove one layer after another by carefully choosing each remedy according to the current totality of symptoms. Each layer initially appears with some insignificant symptoms, which can be difficult to recognize from time to time. Sometimes it takes years before the picture becomes clearer and the correct remedy can be prescribed."

After the removal of the outer layers, it actually did take years before a deeply acting remedy for Eloise could be identified. The key to this remedy was provided by her dreams, in which feelings were expressed which Eloise would not have talked about in such a way. There was this feeling that everything was so strange and peculiar, which she covered up in her daily life with a nervous smile. And then the actual feeling in life of the reserved, timid Eloise, living in a strange, hostile environment in which she is not accepted. This prevailing mood is connected with a special kind of homesickness, a yearning for security which Eloise only experienced on rare occasions with her Amma.

"Homesickness" is one of the key symptoms of the homeopathic remedy *Carbo animalis*. In the records of Samuel Hahnemann, who tested the effects of animal charcoal, as well as that of other substances, on himself and on volunteers, a psychological symptom of this remedy is: "As if abandoned and filled with homesickness. As if in an empty, abandoned city." Another test subject reacted to the dose of animal charcoal with the following emotional state: "Tendency toward loneliness; sad and pensive, she wants only to be alone and avoids any conversation." In homeopathic repertories, the extensive registers of all the symptoms which come from remedy provings and clinical experience, we also find for *Carbo animalis* the feeling that "everything is strange, peculiar." We recognize in these emotional changes fundamental characteristics of Eloise's central feeling in life. Here the potentized animal charcoal is not a remedy for a current physical symptom – it is the cure for severe psychological suffering, which Eloise can first experience herself in the reaction to the remedy. Not until she falls into a severe depression after taking the *Carbo animalis* does it become clear to her that she lived for decades "as if in a dark tunnel," isolated from the world and her surroundings, cut off from life.

"She has the feeling of being absolutely nothing: a non-entity, as though she had no ego inside of her; she believes that others do not take her seriously. But the others actually think that she is a very nice, kind person, very friendly, very generous – and basically a person who will give up her demands." This quote on the psychological state of a *Carbo animalis* person from the *Materia Medica* of Georgos Vithoulkas suits Eloise's soul absolutely perfectly. It is typical for people who need this remedy that they do not participate in life, above all not in social life. They are fighting to survive; for any life beyond this, there is no energy left. This is true of all carbon remedies in homeopathy. In addition to animal charcoal, these consist of wood charcoal, *Carbo vegetabilis*, and the two natural forms of the pure element of carbon: Graphite and Diamond. Carbon and its compounds match homeopathically to people who are afraid of change, who remain in the same situation for years, who play dead out of fear of death and thus appear closer to death than to life. Like Eloise, they can function in daily life when it comes to ensuring their survival or that of their family in their job or at home. But they perform their tasks without pleasure and joy, more like robots.

When they become ill, they often hover between life and death. *Carbo vegetabilis* is indicated in homeopathy in severe illnesses and their final stages, and *Carbo animalis* for cancer in particular. When Eloise dreamed of an incurable disease in her entire body, this was a warning signal for her doctor and an additional indication for *Carbo animalis*. The dramatic reaction then showed what lay dormant in her body. The doctors initially thought that the large abscess which developed in her intestine and later disappeared could be a cancerous tumor.

After the dose of potentiated animal charcoal, the organism came out of its stagnation, awoke from its unreactive state and now tried strenuously to rid itself of old waste products. This type of elimination – which includes the heavy perspiration – can often be seen as an initial reaction to the dose of a homeopathic remedy.

Eloise had to rid herself of old wastes on the psychosocial level as well. Yet this was a longer and more difficult process, which is still in progress today. The process began when her soul came to life after decades of numbness and found its way back out of the dark tunnel into a vivid, colorful world. When she tells today, 10 years later, how she became aware of the trees, the birds and the people around her for the first time, her deep sense of wonder is still perceptible. How she felt herself again, physically, elementally, from one day to the next, and went on to discover and express her own needs; how she went from being a non-entity to a strong, self-confident person after her encounter with her optimal remedy (her *simillimum*) – this transformation is one of the most amazing we have encountered during our work on this book.

As strange and peculiar as this whole story is the similarity between the substance animal charcoal and the fate of little Ellie. Charred ox skin heals the after-effects of severe burns to the body and soul. Is homeopathy so easy? The homeopathic repertories list almost 90 remedies which can be considered for the treatment of burns. *Carbo animalis* is not one of them. And one should not use this case history in the future as a basis for treating the after-effects of burns with *Carbo animalis*. This remedy is only the simillimum when – as was the case with Eloise – the entire picture of her suffering is similar to the remedy picture on all levels.

2. Blessed art thou, Maria!

> *When a man is singing and cannot lift his voice and another comes and sings with him, another who can lift his voice, the first will be able to lift his voice too. That is the secret of the bond between spirits.*
>
> *Martin Buber*

Barbara brings a pile of colorful photo albums, stacks them on the kitchen table and begins to turn the pages: Maria, her fourth child, nursing at the breast as a newborn; Maria having her first bath in the baby tub; Maria with an embroidered pink cap on her thick dark hair, her brothers Thomas and Daniel taking turns holding her. Such a sweet baby. Five thick albums full of photos of Maria. Now she is eleven. A pretty girl with chin-length black curls. Behind the round glasses a curious, bright look in her big brown eyes. She is very proud of the dark blue velvet dress with the purple trim which she wears on special days, and is also proud of her photo albums. "Look," she says, "this is the travel album. Here we were in Turkey. There was a super swimming pool where I still had to hold on at the edge, and here we were on a skiing trip. And this here is full of photos from school. Here you can see my girlfriends, and Thomas when he got his motorcycle. Where are the Christmas pictures, Mama, and the ones with all of the Easter eggs, when we went on a family outing with the church? When I grow up, I want to be a hairdresser. Look, here's a picture where I put up Mama's hair with lots of different barrettes. Shall I show you my new computer? It has lots of new games that I haven't played yet, but I'm already pretty far along with some."

She is trusting, open and more straightforward than many children when she talks to strangers. Whoever watches her swimming and diving can see the blissful expression on her face when she floats in the water, as if weightless, totally entrusting herself to this element. What a happy child, one thinks, when one watches her dive from the board into the pool and go under, straight as an arrow, then float on her back, visibly at ease. Maria's happy disposition comes across so readily.

Her ability to live for the moment is also displayed in her concentration when she counts in her head at breathtaking speed, clapping tens and hundreds in rhythm with her fingers and the palms of her hands and performing calculations. She was the math whiz at her school and in the fourth grade she had only two wrong out of 40 spelling words. Just like the children who go on to the *Gymnasium* (magnet high school). Her handwriting is nice and even. She writes her English vocabulary words neatly on index cards. In physical education she does what she can. The other children let her catch them at dodgeball, since with her slightly jerky movements she is not as agile and quick as her friends. She has her own teacher's aide at school who helps her with the tricky tasks, for example putting the tiny letters back in the reading box, or changing clothes for physical education when she can't undo the small buttons on her jacket fast enough. Her motor coordination is rather far behind that of the others, but her mind can keep up very well.

Maria can now distinctly feel when the darkness, which is just as much a part of her life as the light, threatens to take hold of her. When she can't control the swinging of her head. When her arms jerk as though they didn't belong to her. When the palms of her hands turn outwards and she doesn't know why they are doing this. When she trips and falls over thresholds. When she just can't concentrate anymore, on anything, be it walking, arithmetic or a computer game. When her mind threatens to flee. Then she says, "Mama, I need my medicine." Whether she knows what state she will end up in if she doesn't take her remedy is beyond the borders of our imagination. We only know that at the end, Maria sits doubled up and strangely twisted in front of the mirror, tosses her head back and forth, waves her arms like branches in the wind and makes noises which no longer sound human but more like whimpering, a babbling repetition of a hurdy-gurdy song from deep within, which we do not understand. Then no one can reach her anymore. There sits Maria, the idiot child.

The swinging of her head and arms is the first sign that things are regressing again, if only in small steps at the beginning. Yet the pull into unknown territory cannot be stopped. The return trip back to the mirror. There she sits and searches, perhaps for the other self that she can also be. Maria the pretty, smart and almost completely normal girl. Where and who is Maria? Only the remainder of her cowers in front of the big mirror in the front hall, what is left of something from another world. Can the other Maria recognize herself in this reflection? Perhaps she just can't express it, perhaps she still feels it and is simply caught in this other being. For us "normal people," this dark side is totally strange, a faraway land, which we can reach if at all only through drugs or intoxication. Contorted, rapt, gyrating in unknown spirals. Barbara knows the harbingers of Maria's departure exactly; they are warning signals that send her into a state of terror and panic. Before Maria drifts back into those unknown meanders, she refuses everything that she normally likes to eat. She then accepts only dry bread and tea. As though she were preparing for a long, hard journey.

When Maria was born, Barbara was happy and thankful. Maria was a healthy little girl and her greatest comfort for the stillbirth she had lived through a year before. When they had to take the boy out in the seventh month of pregnancy, Barbara knew already that he was missing both kidneys and had hydrocephalus and spina bifida. He was not capable of surviving and all Barbara had left of him now was a picture in her heart of how the midwife wrapped him in a white cloth and carried him out like a precious treasure. When Barbara soon became pregnant again, she felt a fear gnawing at her whether this child would be healthy. In spite of this, she refused to undergo the amniocentesis urgently recommended by the doctors. Barbara and her husband Johannes are deeply religious people. An abortion would have been fully out of the question for them, even if the child had turned out to be severely handicapped again. And the findings of the ultrasound examinations were indeed alarming. When the girl they had longed for lay in Barbara's arms after a quick and easy birth, it seemed like a miracle. Barbara felt the indescribable grace that a mother experiences when she is given a healthy child after fearing the worst. Johannes fell on his knees next to Barbara's bed and thanked his God. This child was blessed and would thus be called Maria.

The first weeks with Maria were untroubled. The parents proudly returned home with the baby to their two boys, who immediately took her to their hearts. Johannes prayed aloud in the church congregation: "God has given us another child after the death of our Paul. We are so happy that she is healthy and thriving well. How God must love us all!" For months Barbara and Johannes smiled at their little "late bloomer", who did nothing but lie there. What was she waiting for? After six months they slowly began to worry, but they kept this to themselves.

At first glance there is nothing unusual about the photos from Maria's first year. The camera always maintains a certain distance, though. And Maria does not look at the photographer. There is the family picture from her first birthday: on the table, the cake with a big, red candle on top and behind it Maria in the corner of her crib. Standing. Next to it the boys and Papa. What cannot be seen in the photo is that her brother has grabbed her and is holding her up, and there are stiff pillows on either side of her. "It was all contrived," says Barbara. They posed Maria that way because that was how they thought it should be. It looks as though she were standing. As though she could. Actually her ankles were completely twisted and the inner edges of her feet turned upward. The two boys had started walking at 11 and 13 months. Maria couldn't even stand at one year, certainly not on her own. Johannes looks silently at the floor when Barbara confesses, "We never photographed her the way we didn't want to see her; we always made her look better. Looking back it's a pity, because it would be good to see how she really was. She always stared so stiffly, we didn't enjoy photographing her. Her entire body was usually turned back, her chest was twisted, her legs pulled up, her head thrown back. And always this ahmmammam, this wah wah, these horrible sounds. Her arms and hands were always shaking, there was always this rocking motion. It was like that the whole first year. It was dreadful. The twisted hands, the feet turned up, the rocking motion. When I heard these sounds, I knew she wasn't normal and there was nothing we could do about it."

Of course word got around quickly in the small village that after the stillbirth, there was also something wrong with the teacher's fourth child. No one saw Barbara out pushing the carriage like she had with her two boys. Back then, when they were just a few weeks old, the whole family had come to church with the newborns and gone ice skating at the lake festival in the winter when it was almost 20 degrees below zero. But now, even months after the birth, no one saw Barbara outside with the baby. She was afraid of disconcerted glances into the carriage. What should she do at the playground when nine-month-old Maria couldn't crawl and play with the other babies? Crawling was unimaginable, even when the two brothers tirelessly tried to show her how to do it.

Barbara also stayed home with the baby because she was so sickly. In the first months, Maria was almost always ill. She constantly perspired on her neck and the back of her head, so Barbara was afraid of a cool wind. It was worst when Maria slept. Her clothing and bedsheets had to be changed several times in the night because they were soaked with sweat. Bathing was reduced to a minimum. The series of infections didn't let up in spite of all precautions. First a cold, then a cough, then bronchitis. Frequent vomiting. Because Maria didn't cry, she often lay in her vomit, although Barbara got up several times in the night to check on her. Everything was different with her. This wheezing, agonizing cough too, in which the child's shortness of breath could be heard. Nursing the baby was such an effort, nothing like Barbara had experienced with her two sons. Everything took endlessly long and Barbara constantly suffered painful breast infections.

When Maria was six months old and the infections didn't let up, her mother consulted Dr. Swoboda, a physician whom she had come to trust since he had helped her a great deal with her own problems twice. After his first homeopathic prescription, she had finally become pregnant after having only one period a year and a long course of fertility treatments, and had her two boys. Later another homeopathic remedy helped her overcome her seven-year-long eating disorder. Back then she had gone on eating binges after a long phase of anorexia, stuffed everything edible into herself and then vomited everything she ate. When it became clear to her that she had a disorder, she overcame her shame and told her doctor about it. And a few weeks after taking the remedy, she could stop the binging, just like that. Through this type of treatment, Barbara had noticed that she not only became healthy again, but also felt reconnected to her inner strength. Perhaps Dr. Swoboda might know of a good remedy for Maria, so everything would be all right after all.

After his prescription of *Calcarea carbonica*, the susceptibility to colds actually diminished. However, Maria's development didn't proceed – not as Barbara had secretly hoped. She continued just to lie there and didn't move, didn't react to anything, didn't try to grasp anything and didn't follow her mother with her eyes. Her eyes seemed rather to turn more inwards. She became more and more cross-eyed; otherwise nothing changed much. She didn't try making any new sounds; there was no smile of recognition, no movement. She couldn't even turn over. Will she just continue lying there forever, thought Barbara, will I be changing her diapers for the rest of her life? Such thoughts occurred to her more and more frequently and could hardly be repressed. How would it all go on? If Maria was missing all of the normal stages of development, would she end up as a helpless, drooling vegetable in a wheelchair? Was it all right to even think like this? An acquaintance told Barbara to accept the child as she was. Accept her! How was that supposed to be so simple? Today Barbara has long forgiven that childless woman, but back then she would have loved to spit in her face. She continued to hide herself at home with the child. When she was alone, she struggled with her faith. She cried at God, she accused, she pleaded. Why my daughter? Why is fate punishing me again?

But things got even worse. One day, Maria was hanging limply in the infant seat on the kitchen table without paying any attention to the funny puppet hanging over her head, when suddenly her hands jerked up and her entire body was trembling in convulsions, her eyes turned up in her head. Then she was gone. Barbara grabbed the baby out of the seat, shook her, screamed, held her tight in her arms and broke down on her chair. An icy cold took hold of her heart. Finally Maria regained consciousness. Barbara didn't dare to put her child in the car and drive to her homeopath's practice in the city. She called Dr. Swoboda and told him everything that could be important for him to know. Not just the convulsions and subsequent unconsciousness, but also the increasing strabismus, the twisting of Maria's body, the big toe that turned up so absurdly and above all the complete failure to develop.

The next day there was something in the mail for Maria. Three globules were to turn her life around, because three weeks later something totally unexpected happened. Barbara couldn't believe her eyes. Maria must have turned over. But even more astonishing, she was on her hands and knees like a kitten on all fours and was looking through the bars of her crib at her mother. A lively inner radiance shone in her eyes, which Barbara will remember for the rest of her life, and for a moment it took her breath away. Then she lifted her baby out of bed and kissed her from head to toe. If something like this was possible, perhaps more development was in store for Maria after all.

On the advice of their doctor, the parents now consulted the specialists at the large clinic in the capital city. So far they had not dared to take this step. The terrible word epilepsy was uttered. But nothing definitive could be found. In his written report to the family doctor, the specialist stated, "One must say that the cause of this visible and disturbing retardation which points towards an uncertain future is not clear." Little could be expected of further neurological examinations, and professional educational intervention was not necessary, since the parents were already doing everything that was possible. His findings in the 15-month-old child: "No targeted pincer grasp with free index finger, scarcely any building of double syllables, not to mention two-syllable words, exploration only with the mouth. The total impression of the basically friendly child is impaired by the pronounced strabismus. No stable sitting alone, no pulling up to a standing position, can stand on hands and knees only with help." The diagnosis of the specialist, "serious developmental retardation", came along with the prognosis of "a worrying future."

The professor did not know that Maria had not started assuming her unsteady starting position for crawling until just two months before, when she had received the homeopathic remedy. The parents also did not tell him how inactive Maria had been the first thirteen months. They didn't even want to think about what he would have said then. When Barbara and Johannes were home again and the children were all in bed, they sank onto the couch, exhausted, held each other tight and cried the whole night. Everything burst out of them. What they had not admitted to each other for so long. The fears and worries that tormented them. The bitterness. The disappointment. The desperation. What would ever become of their daughter? The professor had made it clear that he couldn't offer them any hope.

Yet Barbara fought. First she stopped hiding herself at home. She made contact with other mothers, even though every time it was a test for her to see how the other children already toddled around on their little legs while her daughter lay there like a beetle stuck on its back. The prognosis of the professor seemed to be confirmed. But her gut feeling told her that the globules had achieved some effect. She tried to recapitulate. Shortly after the dose of the remedy and before Maria got up on her hands and knees, there came a bad cold, a cough with a great deal of mucous, and frequent hiccups. Time and again the child had inhaled very deeply, had cried more than usual and was difficult to calm down. She had also moved more, which Barbara had initially attributed to the fever. At some point Maria had started to sleep very well. Once Barbara thought she distinctly heard Maria shrieking with delight. A first sound of genuine happiness. Was this at all possible? She didn't dare to believe it. But then came the stand on all fours, which made her so happy but was for the professor merely a small indication of normality in an otherwise fully inadequate, abnormal development.

Two months after the sobering examination at the clinic in December, their homeopathic physician decided to give another dose of the potentized water hemlock, Cicuta virosa. Again there was a strong initial reaction: hiccups, perspiration on the neck, vomiting. Once this tumult after the remedy diminished, the positive effect came along about two weeks later. Barbara could later observe this pattern again and again. Yet what she feared most, the convulsions, had already completely disappeared after the first dose.

Over the course of a year, Maria received repeated doses of her globules and her mother kept a log:

On February 11, Maria crawls. A short time later she pulls herself up for the first time on the stair railing. On April 25, after a third dose, Maria can stand alone in the walking frame. In May, she takes her first steps back and forth in the kitchen with her push-along walker. In October of the same year, Maria is given the remedy in a higher potency, C 1,000. Again there is a strong initial reaction, then Maria is able to walk on her own. In November, she is now two years and two months old. She goes exploring through the apartment, chatters in baby talk, piles cans on top of each other, takes everything out of Mama's handbag and beams all over her face with happiness. A few months later, without having spoken any other words, Maria asks her first question. She hears a noise outside and asks, "Who's that coming?" Every time Maria receives her remedy, she takes another leap in her development.

Barbara was very excited when she told the developmental diagnostician in the county seat about Maria's progress. He didn't think much of homeopathy, simply shook his head and didn't want to believe her until he saw it with his own eyes. Barbara could hardly believe it herself. When she first saw Maria standing at the stair railing, on the outer sides of her feet, the soles turned in, she thought, "My God, that looks so awful, she's going to break everything if she tries to walk. How can that possibly work?" But she managed to walk on her deformed feet and they gradually became better.

The diagnostician then wrote very objectively and soberly in his findings on the two-year-old child: "The skew foot has improved in comparison to the last examination. Maria can say Mama, Papa and Baby. She can sing a song. She can eat with a fork by herself. She imitates a great deal, sounds and gestures. She knows all parts of the body. She is learning to undress herself. She is beginning to scribble and paint. She is friendly, but displays a great need for protection. She hears very well. However the muscle tone is reduced on the whole; there is a lack of gross motor coordination." Altogether he estimated the developmental retardation at approximately 30%. At the examination in the large clinic just over a year before, the estimate had been at least 60%. When the diagnostician saw the girl two years later, she was attending kindergarten as an integrated child.

Although she learned a great deal there, a difficult phase began. Her immune system had to struggle with all of the things kindergarten children go through: middle ear infections, colds, childhood diseases. Such illnesses set Maria back more than other children. In these situations, Barbara learned to fear the regression which can still throw her daughter off track today and transport her to the realm where the end of the line is the mirror. Still Maria continued to progress. At the age of four, her motor coordination was much better, but still "inexact." The pediatrician assessed a developmental age of three years in the child with regard to mental capabilities, personal and social development and practical comprehension. So she had caught up some again. At eight years, Maria was the best in her class in arithmetic. And at 11, she achieved the same results on the verbal test as children who went on to the Gymnasium.

What a tireless struggle lay behind it all! It was Barbara who didn't give up. On her own, Maria wouldn't have done it. She wasn't curious by nature; she wouldn't have wanted to learn on her own. And when the pediatrician filled out his report on the four-year-old girl with the trite remark, "Maria has a good vocabulary, is chatty and animated," the inexhaustible dedication of a mother to her child was responsible for this.

She still remembers very well how Maria took her first steps at two-and-a-half, but still didn't speak. Not a single word. And she still hears the accusations of friends and acquaintances that she wasn't doing enough for Maria, although Barbara did spend the whole day singing with her daughter, reciting rhymes and telling her stories. She also remembers the developmental therapist advising her to stimulate the muscles in Maria's mouth with her fingers to get her to utter sounds. But nothing happened.

And then it was homeopathy which provided the next push. The first sentence came. Barbara could have jumped for joy when she saw her daughter standing at the railing saying, "Who's that coming?" Before Maria learned to speak, however, mother and child had to go through a difficult crisis, as is always the case before the next step.

Every dose of the potentized poisonous plant first hurled Maria into the purgatory of initial aggravation. Barbara still looks back today with horror at the terrible eczema which broke out on the palms of her daughter's hands and the soles of her feet in suppurating pustules for almost six weeks. In a New Year's Eve photo from that time, a very pale, tired-looking Maria can be seen under garlands and streamers. She felt terrible back then, emotionally as well. She already started screaming in pain when Barbara tried to pull her pants down over her infected feet.

Barbara slept as little as Maria, for at night she held the whimpering child in her arms and let Maria run her infected hands through Barbara's hair, and endured the incessant whining and screaming until morning, when Maria finally dozed off, exhausted.

This went on for six weeks, and then mother and child were rewarded with the next developmental step. The rash disappeared and Maria began to speak. One year later she stood for the first time on skis, supported by Papa. After such hard-fought successes, Barbara often had to think of the day her little girl had her first seizure and lay there limp in her arms, as if she were dead. And now Maria on skis? Oh yes, everything came late, came with effort, certainly not on its own. Whether it was learning to eat alone, to use the toilet, to walk or to speak. But Barbara was endlessly thankful that it came at all, she was thankful for every step and she had faith that the progress would continue.

Her Maria is truly blessed. She has a doctor who found the correct remedy for her. She lives in the country, in a village where life is slower than in other places. Her parents have been able to provide optimal conditions for their handicapped child. Here they have received completely unbureaucratic support from the community. Barbara and her husband are both teachers at the school in their village and are very involved in the church. Maria was assigned a remedial teacher in kindergarten and later in school she had her own teacher's aide. Those with handicapped children know how important special approvals can be. It is thus no problem for Maria to arrive at school an hour later. Like many developmentally delayed children, she needs twelve hours of sleep and a lot of time for getting up and dressed. The teaching methods in a normal school are also often not sufficient for such a child. Barbara took Montessori training so she can give her child supplemental instruction at home with a different method than in school, as she has observed that Maria learns best through her sense of touch.

Maria's first tries at writing were nonetheless wide of the mark. As a teacher, Barbara had never seen a pupil who wrote such twisted letters. From A to Z, they lay totally scribbled on their backs, far more complicated than they actually were. Through tactile exercises and with the keys of the computer, Maria finally did learn to write. Her first letter was sent in its original form to her homeopathic doctor. A copy is mounted in Maria's photo album: "Mama should stay healthy, Papa should stay healthy, Mama cleans the house, Your Maria." It was her first free writing, not just copying letters as she had done until then. Maria formulated it without help.

This first letter was a surprise like everything else. At first Barbara thought her daughter was only joking when she asked for paper. She didn't think she was capable back then. And two years later when Maria corrected her mother's spelling of a word and was right, it was her mother who nearly had a seizure. She laughed and laughed until she had to gasp for air and the tears were streaming down her face.

Maria could already read when she started school. And she worked with her mother on the other subjects before they came up in school. Barbara tried to prevent Maria from feeling pressured in school, since she was always slower than the others. When she taught Maria arithmetic, she wondered how they would deal with hundreds, as Maria was just able to handle the tens and the numbers from 1 to 99 with her fingers and hands. Then Barbara stumbled upon the cybernetic method, which a German mathematician had developed for his own child. Maria thus learned arithmetic with number packets, in keeping with the natural tactile talent of primary school pupils. Barbara was always afraid that the teacher and the other pupils might close in on their lead, for she knew that under stress her daughter would quickly confuse everything she had learned.

Cicuta was like a learning aid for Maria. After each dose she could concentrate better again. She drew and painted much more exactly and easily, read more attentively and could do mental arithmetic even faster. When the effect wore off, her arithmetic slowed down, she forgot words, she began to trip and stagger and ultimately drifted into her other world. Barbara knows that Maria could only achieve all of her accomplishments because she was helped from morning until night. While Maria pinned up her mother's hair, she unconsciously trained her fine motor skills by handling the small clips and barrettes. At the same time Mama quizzed her on spelling words, or had her recite the multiplication tables, in order to train her concentration and the interaction of both brain hemispheres. During the school vacations, she reviewed all of the subject material with Maria. For the first time during the last vacation though, she didn't do any schoolwork with Maria. She wanted a vacation for herself for once, even though she was afraid that the multiplication tables might be gone again. No, it is not good for her to think of all the precious time she spent teaching her them.

Maria still has no official diagnosis, there is no metabolic disorder and her EEG's are normal. No one knows what disease Maria has or what the deficit which she suffers from is called. When Barbara had to wait especially long the last time for the preparation of the next higher potency of *Cicuta*, she was desperate, because she knows how far away Maria can drift. Maria knows it too and pleaded, "Mama, please give me *Cicuta*." She could feel that she wasn't well. She was tired, clumsy and no longer believed she was capable of anything. And they had to keep waiting and watching how Maria suffered and continued to go downhill, unable to reach the level she had been on before. *Cicuta* still helped her in the old potency for more ordinary problems such as colds or a bladder infection. But it didn't reach as deeply to her central disturbance anymore. Not until she received a higher potency did she begin to move forward again.

She has taken a big step out into the world. Now she feels confident enough to call friends and play with them outside on her own. Without Mama. On the big lot in front of the old factory, Maria rides on her new red scooter and romps around for hours with the neighbors' children.

Before she goes out to meet her friends, she hugs Mama and Papa affectionately and doesn't want to stop kissing them. She doesn't have the emotional distance that other children her age slowly develop. Barbara is worried about this, since Maria's breasts are developing and she will soon enter puberty. What if someone takes advantage of her innocence? How will she continue to manage in school? Will she really be able to become a hairdresser one day? Barbara doesn't believe it yet. How will Maria ever be able to wind fine strands of hair on tiny perm curlers? She has gotten through primary school, which didn't seem possible at the beginning. And Barbara will think of a new method for dealing with secondary school. She is already working on it. But without *Cicuta* it won't work. In spite of all of her effort and support, even Barbara, the tireless fighter for her child, would not be able to protect Maria from that frightening state without the remedy: when she kneels in front of the mirror, tosses her head back and forth, waves her arms and utters the sounds that come from that other dark and nameless world which is beyond our comprehension.

Commentary

When Maria was brought to the homeopathic physician Dr. Swoboda in her first year, there was no long biography of a life full of changes to report and Maria was not able to describe her subjective complaints herself. With infants and small children, the homeopath must rely primarily on his own observation and that of the parents. The prescription of a remedy in this phase of life is often based on only a few symptoms which are, moreover, not highly specific to the sick individual. This lack of individualization necessary for successful homeopathic treatment is compensated for by the fact that children generally tend to react to the subtle stimuli of this medicine more sensitively than adults. Even a less than optimal remedy can thus lead to a cure especially in acute illnesses.

The same cannot be said, however, for disease processes which are deeply rooted in the congenital and acquired constitution of a person, in his physical and mental structure. In such cases for children and adults, one must find the most suitable homeopathic remedy, a so-called "constitutional remedy", which covers not only the current symptoms, but also the entire recognizable condition of the organism, its special way of reacting, its weak points, its peculiarities. Recurring infections such as those Maria suffered, as well as developmental delays, are among the most frequent problems requiring constitutional homeopathic treatment in pediatric practice.

When Maria was six months old, her parents simply thought their nearly motionless, passive baby was a "late bloomer." Her failure to develop at this age was nonetheless taken into consideration for the remedy selection. This very symptom, together with the tendency toward infections and the pronounced head sweating during sleep, clearly pointed in the direction of *Calcarea carbonica Hahnemannii*. This remedy, which is often indicated in infancy, was certainly effective as a constitutional remedy in Maria's case, since it not only cured the acute respiratory infection, but also her general susceptibility to infections. However, the potentized lime of the oyster shell was obviously unable to reach the deep layer where the problem of the delayed development lay, virtually "programmed." The parents thus waited in vain for their child to grasp objects, turn over, crawl or babble.

Finally Maria herself sent a dramatic signal that something had to be done. The seizure demanded stronger homeopathic action. When the possible remedies in this situation are listed with the help of a repertory according to the Law of Similars and the combination of Maria's characteristic symptoms, it is interesting to note that most of these remedies are derived from highly poisonous substances. The fly agaric is among them, as is the poisonous secretion of the toad Bufo vulgaris or the sap from the capsules of the opium poppy. From the homeopathic point of view, a remedy for Maria's disease picture needs to be capable of triggering such a threatening state in a healthy person. *Cicuta virosa* fits this description and is one of the main remedies for treating seizures. If someone takes just a single gram of the fresh root of the water hemlock, he will die within one hour of violent convulsions which seize the entire body. The deadly effect is absolutely certain, and after just a short time, the poison cannot be detected in the bloodstream.

The poisoning symptoms of Cicuta and many other highly toxic substances form the basis for their use in homeopathy. The highly diluted and potentized water hemlock is thus indicated for epileptic seizures with subsequent unconsciousness, as they occur in Cicuta poisoning. The most important source of information for the homeopath, however, is the proving of the potentized substances on healthy persons. In one such remedy proving, Samuel Hahnemann already noted of a test person who had taken a diluted tincture of Cicuta: "When walking she does not tread properly on the soles of the feet; they tip over towards the inside." And Vithoulkas adds to this symptom: "Walks on the outer edge of the foot." To the proving and poisoning symptoms are added the clinical observations made on patients after the use of a particular remedy. An especially precise observer was the famous American physician James Tyler Kent, whose repertory has been indispensable for many generations of homeopaths. In his standard work, only six remedies are listed for the symptom "Strabismus convergens" (eyes turned inward), with *Cicuta virosa* emphasized in boldface type. And in his Lectures on Materia Medica, Kent notes among other observations about the water hemlock: "Sweat on the scalp when sleeping. Child rolls head from side to side."

If one examines the list of symptoms of *Cicuta virosa* compiled from the poisoning picture, the remedy proving and observations of patients, all of the essential disease phenomena we know from Maria's story can be found: the seizures with unconsciousness, the strabismus, the markedly skew feet and also the central problem. Because in the Synthesis Repertory, a modern expansion of Kent's listing of symptoms, *Cicuta* is listed as one of the most important remedies for developmental standstill in children. In the face of such a strong agreement, also of the rare and characteristic symptoms, a reaction to the potentized water hemlock could certainly be anticipated. However, the degree of this reaction exceeded the expectations of the parents and probably of the homeopath as well. Most important at first, of course, was that no more seizures occurred. Maria was thus saved from the stigma of epilepsy and the long-term medication therapy normally associated with it. And her vital force could now unfold as it should after some delay.

One step after another, she caught up, according to the sequence laid out by nature. The motor development of a person always follows the same pattern from the head downwards to the feet. Every child learns to control his muscles from top to bottom. First he is capable of controlling his head before he can use his shoulders, arms and hands voluntarily. The development then moves down the back and hips to the legs, until the child finally learns to walk. This capability is innate and the natural development processes and their sequence can hardly be influenced externally. The task of the parents during motor development is therefore limited to providing space for movement, encouraging their child and recognizing and praising him for his progress. For Maria, the normal program never got started and Barbara and Johannes were thus unable to offer her support.

All of this changed after *Cicuta*. Yet what right do we have to attribute this reversal in Maria's life to the homeopathic treatment?

We do not know how she would have developed without the influence of the water hemlock. We also cannot compare Maria's fate to that of other developmentally delayed children who later end up in wheelchairs and special homes. After all, it happens to be a fundamental characteristic of homeopathy that every sick person must be viewed individually. This is what makes it so difficult to evaluate the successes of this medicine with the statistical methods of conventional medicine in randomized double-blind studies, because in these objective studies, importance is placed on eliminating subjective influences on the participants as much as possible. An objective, "inter-individual" comparison with other children who are also developmentally delayed is not possible with case histories. Yet Maria's history offers us the special opportunity for "intra-individual" comparison. We can readily judge the influence of the remedy on her over the years by seeing what happens when the effect wears off again, when things reach the point where Maria says, "Mama, please give me *Cicuta*".

Then she can no longer concentrate, becomes clumsy and loses control of her body and mind. She regresses, returns to a much earlier phase of her life, becomes a babbling infant again. The astonishing similarity between the remedy picture of Cicuta virosa and Maria's disease picture is also displayed in this process, as the theme of regression is also mentioned in the remedy proving of the water hemlock. In his Materia Medica Pura from the year 1819, Samuel Hahnemann describes the following symptom of an adult test person: "He felt like a child of seven or eight years old, objects were very dear and attractive to him, as toys are to a child." And Georgos Vithoulkas writes of *Cicuta*: "In chronic disease states with mental and emotional effects, the symptoms of immaturity and the childlike, even childish nature are apparent. Sometimes the patients make a completely innocent impression." The last sentence also describes Maria's nature in her good phases, when she has taken her remedy and is alert again, with improved motor skills and attentiveness during her daily tasks. For ten years Maria and her parents have known the effect of her remedy and are building their hopes on it.

This effect – and this is a fundamental criterion for the success of a remedy – has been reliably reproduced over all of this time.

With one exception. After several doses of the same potency, the effect becomes exhausted. This is a well known phenomenon in homeopathy. In such a case, the same remedy is given in a higher potency. Proceeding from the 200 C, for which the mother tincture of the fresh water hemlock root was diluted and succussed 200 times in a ratio of 1:100, the potency was raised in Maria's case to 1,000 C (= 1M), then to 10,000 C (=XM) and finally to 100,000 C (=CM). It is one of the riddles of homeopathy that these infinite dilutions work at all, and often even better than the low potencies, and that there is apparently no natural upper limit for potentizing. In practice, however, the time and effort increases with the level of the potency, so that an infinite increase is not possible. At any rate, some common homeopathic remedies have been potentized up to the level of 1,000,000 C (=MM).

What will happen to Maria if *Cicuta* CM no longer works and the scale of high potencies has been exhausted because no higher potency of the water hemlock exists? One can then –and Dr. Swoboda has done this already – change to a different form of preparation, for example to the so-called Q or LM potencies, which are diluted 1:50,000 at each potency step. Maria is continuing to progress with this form. Yet it was not certain how she would react to it. In this respect, statistics are of no use to us in homeopathy. We are just as uncertain about how long Maria will continue to need her remedy. Since she has needed it for so long and in repeated doses, this shows how deeply the problem is rooted in her constitution. We are not able to determine where this problem comes from, which gene or which phase of embryonic development is involved, as in so many cases of delayed childhood development. However in homeopathy, the medicine of similarity between disease and remedy, there is a clear diagnosis for Maria's illness. It is *Cicuta virosa*.

3. The End of the Line

> *All that I have and possess, you have given all that to me. I now give it back to you, O Lord. Give me your love and your grace, for that is enough for me.*
>
> Ignatius von Loyola

"Ruth has suicidal thoughts," said Ingeborg on the telephone. What ever gave her that idea? Nonsense! Mama would never kill herself. Claudia was convinced of that. Her mother was far too religious to think of committing suicide. And she was a strong woman who never got depressed. Anyhow that was what she always said. Claudia had phoned Ruth's best friend because of her mother's upcoming 60th birthday and Ingeborg had then shared her observations. She had the feeling that Ruth was not doing well at all. Claudia couldn't understand this feeling. Ruth was the same as always. Balanced. Relatively healthy. She worked at lot and often talked about the company. How hard everything was these days. Claudia had also heard Mama's friends and acquaintances complaining about bad business conditions. Most of them were business people. Complaining a little was perfectly normal for them.

Claudia got along well with her mother. They could talk openly with each other. So Claudia knew how Ruth felt about depression. It was a much-discussed topic in the family, as Ruth's mother had suffered from depression her whole life. And her cousins as well.

So severe that she was no longer able to take care of her children and had to spend long periods of time in the clinic. Although she was physically healthy and free of financial worries, with a husband she could depend on, she sat in the black recesses of her soul, locked in and trapped, where no light, affection, sympathy or loving words could reach her. Mama empathized deeply with her. Yet at the same time she saw in this depression a certain ingratitude towards life and towards God. She felt that you just had to tackle things and hold your own. The rest would fall into place, somehow.

Her father would surely have come back after the war, after he had deserted and gone to France. If only Alma, her mother, hadn't been so fainthearted. That was what Ruth thought, and she often told Claudia about it. An insatiable longing for her father always remained with her. But she could understand that he wanted to live. He simply couldn't bear his anxious and deeply sad wife anymore.

Oh yes, it was hard back then, when Ruth and her siblings and her mother Alma stood before the ruins of their town house in eastern Germany when the war was over. Nothing was left. The beautiful old furniture, Alma's jewelry and furs, father's study. Everything was burned up. Ruth's enormous room with all of her dolls as well. Her childhood suddenly lay there in rubble and ashes. It was a shock. She was six years old. But still, others had to live through the same thing. And they didn't cry for the rest of their lives at an empty table like Alma. Ruth never saw her father again. And she blamed her mother for this. She swore to herself that she would never capitulate. And she stuck it out, even when she had to bury her romantic childhood dreams of true love and a happy home bit by bit in her daily life.

After the telephone call, Claudia talked to her older sister Dorothea about Mama. She hadn't noticed anything unusual about her either. She was like always, she said, stubborn in her own way and sometimes a little tired. But no wonder. After all, she had been working for almost forty years and would soon be celebrating her 60th birthday. The preparations, the invitations, the seating of the guests; it was all an effort for her. And Dorothea's separation from her husband was surely stressful for her mother as well. Ruth didn't hold it against her daughter that the marriage had failed. Things hadn't gone any better for her. Papa had left her for another woman after 26 years of marriage. She was almost fifty then.

When that happened, she fell into a real slump. Claudia can still picture her mother lying for days on the chaise longue out on the veranda, a magazine spread open on her lap which she didn't read, her empty gaze fixed straight ahead of her. Claudia was preparing back then to study abroad. Every time she looked out of her window towards the veranda, she saw Mama lying there, still and immovable. As though she were on vacation. Yet vacation was a foreign word for Ruth. Her husband's business had always had priority in her life. She had been the boss there. Now she wore the same old pants every day, the ones she normally wore only on weekends when she worked in the garden. Yet she didn't even care anymore about the flower beds and plants that had been her pride and joy. Claudia talked to her again and again about her mood, sat down next to her, asked, waited. But Mama was uncommunicative. She just needed a little time, she said. Claudia shouldn't even consider changing her plans. And so she went to England for a year.

When Claudia returned, Ruth already had everything under control again. With some inheritance money she had bought her own business. The field was new for her. But why shouldn't she be able to sell lingerie and corsetry if she had sold leather goods and riding boots in Papa's company? The main thing was being able to stand on her own feet, independent of her ex-husband; she didn't want to fight with him over the alimony she was legally entitled to. Her store didn't make her rich. But it supported her, two saleswomen and an apprentice. And it allowed her to resume the life she had led as a businesswoman. Claudia was happy that Ruth was her old self again.

This did not suit Dorothea, however. She had often reproached her mother for not taking better care of her and Claudia. Business, business, business. There was never anything else. The daughters were there in the background and had to go with the flow until Ruth pushed them out of the nest as soon as possible. "It didn't do you any harm," was Mama's view of the situation. She had to become an adult at 18 and her children could certainly do the same. And now that Dorothea was standing with her back to the wall with her twins, Mama was letting her down again. Instead of fulfilling her duties as a grandmother, she only thought about her business.

As understanding as Ruth was otherwise, she could not handle criticism very well. She was not willing to accept the accusation that her business activities had led her to neglect her duties as a mother. She had always done her best. For the business and for the children. And that was that! Neither of the women was willing to give in, and the dispute poisoned the atmosphere between mother and daughter.

Ruth didn't show anyone how this conflict gnawed at her. She kept on going. What else should she have done? She wasn't used to anything else. And all of her capital was tied up in the business. Working less was not an option. So she continued to drive to the store every morning at eight o'clock and home again at eight o'clock in the evening, did her housework and went to bed, also on Saturdays. She could rest only when she slept.

Until one day she could no longer sleep because of worries about her business. Every night she lay awake and brooded. She estimated her stock and the personnel costs against the outstanding debts and calculated the turnover for the next year. Would it have to be 25, 30 or 50 percent higher in order for her to pay off her debts? It was hopeless. An increase was unimaginable in any case.

More and more she saw herself on the verge of bankruptcy. Yet she kept her financial worries carefully hidden from her friends and family. She asked her suppliers for payment deferrals and warned her customers about their overdue bills. She kept a stiff upper lip, talked until she was blue in the face in order to sell more, listened, empathized, related to everyone's troubles. But even with personal involvement and individual attention, she wasn't able to retain her customers. Expensive silk lingerie was no longer in demand. And at the department store everything was cheaper. She had no strength or ideas left for modern marketing strategies, clever advertising or developing a new clientele. Her energy was gone, as if it had been drained away. Her thoughts now constantly revolved around her problems in the business. If she wanted to get another loan from the bank, she would have to put up her small house as collateral, the only retirement benefit she had. If she didn't borrow any money, she couldn't pay her employees anymore. Leave the others in the lurch in order to save herself from imminent poverty? She didn't really have any choice. Her ruin seemed inevitable.

She was exhausted to the limit of her emotional will to survive. As hard as she tried, she couldn't find a solution. The thoughts that constantly turned in her head paralyzed her and sapped her strength. In the mornings she was afraid to begin the day, afraid of looking people in the eye. This feeling of being totally helpless and without any hope was not completely new to her. Her mother and her cousins must have felt very much the same. Ruth fought desperately, but it just didn't work anymore. She, who always radiated optimism and drive, had to admit to herself that she had failed. In order to keep up appearances, she had obviously gotten in way over her head. A fraud, that was what she was. Everyone was supposed to see how well she could get something off the ground on her own. She had also wanted to see it and prove it to herself. Now it was clear: she couldn't do it. She would soon fail at everything that was important to her in life. And everyone would see. Nothing could be done. And she and she alone was to blame for this misfortune.

How often did Ruth pick up the phone to call Claudia? Yet every time, she hung up again at the last minute. She didn't want to burden her daughter. But who could she bare her soul to? Among all of her good friends, there was no one she felt she could open up to. Some had depended on Ruth's strength and had come to her with their problems. The others were solid and successful in life. She felt too ashamed of herself to approach them. Ruth absolutely did not want to lose face. So she pulled herself together during the day and cried quietly into her pillow at night, so the neighbors wouldn't hear her sobs through the thin walls.

Her only confidant was the wood carving of the archangel Gabriel in her bedroom. She tried to pray as she had always done, "Lord, help me. I pray to you in my hour of need!" Throughout her life, prayer had been the source of her strength. But now she couldn't find it inside of her. It was as if everything were dead. A new packet of sleeping pills lay on the night table. Go to sleep and never wake up again. It was certainly a big temptation. But even in her darkest hours, Ruth never seriously considered this solution.

Her desperation finally did find a way to express itself. More and more often, her face swelled up overnight and took on a bloated appearance, without contours. In the morning she was completely disfigured. Looked like a monster. She went for allergy tests. But nothing unusual was found besides the hay fever she already knew about and a tendency towards an asthmatic cough. When she touched her swollen face with her fingers in the morning, she didn't want to look in the mirror. Ruth bought herself a large pair of sunglasses and a cortisone cream to hide and combat her disfigured face. She would get through her birthday party this coming Saturday and call an emergency meeting at her business in the week after. Her employees finally had to be informed.

At the birthday party it was an effort for her to play the role of the radiant grandmother and successful businesswoman. Claudia could see how delighted she was at the performances her grandchildren gave. But Claudia also saw how Mama fell apart when she thought no-one was looking. And she saw in her face the incredible effort she made not to lose control of herself.

When Claudia called her two days later, Ruth's voice was as thin and fragile as glass. A bad cold, I didn't sleep so well, nothing serious. Until Claudia said, "Mama, that's enough now." Then Ruth burst into tears. She had fallen on the street on her way home. Her legs had simply buckled under her, just like that, for no reason. She fell to the ground and wasn't able to get up again.

Her feeling was, "I am paralyzed!" Something terrible and unimaginable had attacked her. The command that her head gave to the lower half of her body didn't reach her legs. They remained weak, without strength. There was only this great, absolute powerlessness in her. Only fragments of thoughts, "at the end of my rope," "I can't do it," "It's not me."

Someone pulled her up on her feet. She tried to bring her rising panic under control by taking concentrated breaths. Everything around her was a blur. Houses, streets, people. Even time. Somehow she dragged herself to her car. How long it took and how she did it, she doesn't remember. Then she found herself in her bed. And there she was flooded by a nameless fear, the feeling of being completely incapable of moving, an endless weakness. She stayed in bed, heavy, as if crushed, without any strength. In the morning, when Claudia called, she suddenly remembered the speechless, shaken expressions on the faces of her employees after the emergency meeting at her business. They simply couldn't believe how serious the situation was. Although she herself was close to a breakdown. Ruth didn't know how to go on. Still her daughter had difficulty convincing her to finally seek medical assistance.

When Claudia left her mother in the examining room – she insisted on being alone with the doctor – Ruth sat in the patient's chair looking as weak and helpless as a baby bird that had fallen from the nest. This scene reminded Claudia of one of the few situations from her childhood when she had seen her mother cry. Back then Mama had had all four wisdom teeth extracted. Her jaw was thick and swollen and tears were streaming down her face. It was just a brief glimpse behind the strong armor to a completely different woman, who was also her mother: weak, sensitive and in need of support. Why hadn't they ever seen this?

Even now, Ruth didn't ask for help - she gave the homeopathic physician a clear order. She had to be at the store the next day and therefore expected fast and effective treatment. Without bringing up for the time being how she felt deep down inside, she first reported to him only what she saw as essential and began with the sudden attack of paralysis the evening before. She wasn't yet conscious of the fact that in this scene, a fundamental pattern of her life was depicted. Perhaps it had all started with the fact that she had to grow up very quickly. Although she was still a child herself in the years after the war, she took over increasing responsibility for her younger siblings and the cousins who had become war orphans. She earned money for the family as a young girl and was forced to forego university studies because her depressive mother could not survive on her own and needed her support. Then, in the business owned by her husband and parents-in-law, she constantly had to prove through her work over two decades that she was worthy of this family. As hard as she tried, it was never enough. On top of that, her scheming mother-in-law persecuted her with relentless hate and growing jealousy. After the divorce, her husband's entire family once again regarded Ruth as the "nobody" she had been when she married into the business.

In this difficult phase too, her old survival strategy prevailed: persevere, fight, be strong. She bought the lingerie store against the advice of experts in order to demonstrate that she could manage entirely on her own.

"I really wanted to find out for myself," she told the doctor, "and now I know that I can't do it. I wanted to get something off the ground myself."

"And now your legs don't carry you anymore. How did you feel when you suddenly couldn't walk anymore?"

"All of my strength was drained out of me. But I didn't want to lie there on the street and be taken to the hospital by strangers. I wanted to walk myself. I know, I have to do it myself, but I don't know how I should do it."

"You don't have to. You don't have to be strong."

With these words, the doctor finished the patient interview, which had actually probed much deeper than Ruth had intended. And these last words, as trite and simple as they might sound, have accompanied her ever since.

It was the first time that someone allowed her to let go and granted her the right to be weak.

It was like an absolution for her and it came with the single dose of five globules of the homeopathic remedy *Ignatia*. That evening she took the remedy after a quick prayer, "Lord, I can't do it, you do it!" That night, Ruth slept deeply and well without sleeping pills for the first time in months and woke up the next morning without her paralyzing fear of the day - and without a swollen face! With the new realization, "I don't have to," it was not difficult for her to go to her store. The figures there were still in the red and the situation wasn't rosy, but Ruth's perspective had changed somehow. She could take action again and was now increasingly willing to ask for and accept support from others. Slowly, she could almost feel her old strength returning to her body.

After two weeks she felt strong enough to call the family together, bluntly reveal her situation and take the necessary consequences. After discussions with a financial adviser, she was able to cut costs and put her store back on its feet through layoffs and a move to smaller premises. On a reduced scale, she continued to run her business for seven years before handing it over without losses and with a good name.

Her homeopathic remedy became her constant companion. Whenever she felt ill or incapable of coping with a situation, she took *Ignatia* for a few days. It worked for common colds as well as for allergic asthma. Even the pain and other complaints after a vein operation were relieved by the same remedy. *Ignatia* also helped her through times of mourning associated with death and separation, for Ruth was confronted more than others in life with the loss of loved ones. And whenever the old pattern of feeling overwhelmed and burdened by financial worries broke through again, this remedy was her refuge and salvation. She has never again reached the point she was at when she lay on the street with paralyzed legs, unable to go any farther. For she has learned to take better care of herself and take more time for herself. When she is worried and fearful, she doesn't hide it anymore. She can open up to others. With assured self-confidence, Ruth trusts in her strengths today, such as her special sense of humor, her keen ability to empathize and her great inner peace, which can be felt by the people around her. Towards her friends and family, she radiates a deep, serene wisdom and calmness.

Commentary

Ruth sought homeopathic help in an acute crisis situation. Her very existence seemed so threatened to her that she even thought of suicide. The central problem in her life had been compressed into one moment: she was on the ground and could not get up again on her own. Almost like a role-play, her organism staged this paralysis out on the street and thus expressed her dilemma in a graphic way. It couldn't be concealed anymore - she was ruined. In this scenario lies the key to understanding this person and her remedy.

Although ostensibly simply a crisis intervention, this case demonstrates the technique of homeopathic case analysis with the help of a repertory. In the first step, the essential components of the key scenario must be identified. Here the objective facts are not as important for the homeopath as the subjective experience of the patient in this critical situation. She is not really paralyzed, even though she has the feeling that she cannot move her legs. The first symptom that was looked up in the repertory was therefore: "Delusion, she cannot walk."

The term "delusion" in the repertories refers not only to particular symptoms of mental illness, but also in general to any type of one-sided or distorted subjective perception. If Ruth had really been paralyzed, one would have had to study the rubrics dealing with paralysis of the extremities.

In addition, the background of her inability to move, namely the feeling of being ruined and close to bankruptcy, belongs to the category of subjective perception. The homeopath couldn't assess her business situation, of course, but he could recognize an important element of her state in the intensity of her fear. For this reason he also chose for the case analysis the rubric "Delusion, she is ruined." Later developments then showed that this feeling did not completely reflect reality. Otherwise she could not have run her business for seven more years.

What else does Ruth feel when she is lying on the ground, incapable of doing anything? She is ashamed of her incapability because she believes it is her fault. The corresponding rubrics in the repertory are "Reproaches himself" and "Ailments from shame."

As with delusions, there are also numerous entries in the "Mind" chapter under "Ailments from..." - such as from shock, grief, anger, jealousy. These rubrics point to the emotional weaknesses of a person, to his special sensitivity and vulnerability in a certain area. *Ignatia* thus reacts especially strongly to situations associated with shame. However, we also find this remedy in rubrics such as "Ailments from loss of position"; "Ailments from business failure"; or "Ailments from wounded honor."

In the remedy picture of *Ignatia*, the characteristic traits of Ruth's state of mind at the time of the key homeopathic scenario can thus be clearly recognized. It is the only remedy which completely covers the epitome of the symptoms of this moment. Nevertheless, its significance for this patient goes beyond the acute crisis intervention.

Ignatia is often used in homeopathy as a so-called grief remedy for severe psychological stress, especially when the patient tends towards hysterical reactions such as crying fits, trembling of the entire body, fainting spells or, as in this case, symptoms of paralysis. James Tyler Kent made the observation which became so important for Ruth, "*Ignatia* heals a very particular type of paralysis, namely temporary hysterical paralysis." It is very typical that such reactions, which vary in severity up to a nervous breakdown, occur in a situation of being totally overwhelmed. At some point the woman – *Ignatia* is mainly indicated in women – sees no escape and is overwhelmed by her feelings. Before she reaches this point, however, she has often fought for many years to assert herself and her ideals, to live up to her own high standards, and has neglected her own emotional needs in the process.

The contemporary American homeopath Catherine Coulter writes of the *Ignatia* woman, "She may make a supreme effort to appear carefree, so as not to burden others with her sorrow. Thus, while *Ignatia* is easily recognized in the grieving individual, it is also indicated for the overtly "cheerful" (Boenninghausen) one, as well as the reserved, non-communicative one who keeps her troubles to herself but continues to brood."

In this compensated state of the *Ignatia* woman, no trace of hysteria can be detected, no ostentatious sobbing, no dramatic outbursts. When she suffers, she doesn't let it show. The characteristic rubric in the repertory for this side of Ignatia is *Silent grief*. As long as women like Ruth bear their pain quietly, they will not go to the doctor. They do not seek help until after a breakdown. Then it is important to find the typical behavior pattern of *Ignatia* in the history of the current crisis. It belongs to the hysterical paralysis like the other side of a coin. Because it ran in Ruth's case like a thread through her life, *Ignatia* became her personal remedy, a constitutional remedy, which was later able to help her through various physical and emotional problems. In her case it is a remedy for her as a whole, with her individual weaknesses and typical patterns of reaction.

A holistic, constitutional match on these lines tends to be the exception in the homeopathic application of the St. Ignatius bean. In practice, it is frequently used regardless of the biographical background, when a person is overwhelmed by pain and grief, usually caused by a great loss. This can be a death, disappointed love, financial ruin, job dismissal or social decline. When people don't know how to go on, are completely desperate and believe all is lost, many react in a very similar way, independent of their individual traits. For this reason it is sometimes acceptable in acute homeopathic prescribing to deviate from the strict principle that a similar remedy must be selected according to characteristic individual criteria.

This also applies to other situations in which personal traits move into the background and various people react in a similar way, for example in the course of a flu epidemic. Here those affected can display very similar symptoms and therefore need the same homeopathic remedy. Other examples of uniform reaction patterns are sudden shock experiences or physical injuries such as bruises or a concussion. Remedies such as *Opium* or *Arnica* have often been useful in such cases, leading practitioners to speak of "proven indications". Because prescriptions based on the present situation and not on the constitution of a person do not require a great deal of homeopathic experience and can still produce astonishing effects, these offer beginners the best introduction to homeopathy and are entirely acceptable for emergency treatment. Profound cures such as Ruth's, however, can only be expected when the remedy for an acute problem is identical to the constitutional remedy.

4. Lovesick

> *They loved each other because everything around them willed it, the trees and the clouds and the sky over their heads and the earth under their feet. Perhaps their surrounding world, the strangers they met in the street, the landscapes drawn up for them to see on their walks, the rooms in which they lived or met, were even more pleased with their love than they were themselves.*
>
> Boris Pasternak

Lara. We shall call her Lara. After Larissa Fjodorowna, Doctor Zhivago's love. For she had yearned for such a love all of her life. A love that seldom exists in reality and one that is so poignantly described by Boris Pasternak. For our Lara, the room where they met is in a big German city, in the apartment of the man she is devoted to, for whom she neglects everything – her profession, her family, herself. The man who is the object of her deep yearning for love looks like the man of her dreams: he is tall, dark, slender. Like Omar Sharif as Yuri Zhivago. Lara is crazy about him.

It was a romantic place where they met for the first time. A place where amorous play between the sexes fills the atmosphere and still remains only a suggestion or possibility. A dance school, where classical and Latin-American dances are practiced by couples who do not know each other in their daily lives. Dances where they touch each other, find their rhythm together, where the woman must let the man lead: tango, rumba, slow foxtrot. Lara doesn't go there because she wants to meet a new man after her divorce, but because she passionately loves to dance. She loves this delicate and at the same time distant play, the harmony between strangers, adapting to the new partner, the touch and the mutual concentration on the rhythm of the music.

Lara feels someone's gaze fixed on her. The man who is watching her appears to have everything she finds attractive in a man. He has striking features, is perfectly dressed and seems humorous and cultivated. She doesn't let it show that he has aroused her interest. "No one wants you anyway," her father had told his little girl again and again. Like a curse, this remark still haunts the adult woman. So she remains in the role that she enjoys playing for others. Cool, collected, disciplined. Her severe pantsuits reveal nothing about her childhood dreams. She is not sure. Does she really have enough interest in him? Perhaps it is not worth giving up her distance.

But then he approaches her. He not only starts the game but goes beyond that, narrowing more and more boldly the space she keeps between them. He works her over, pulling all the stops. Flowers, opera tickets, lavish invitations to dinner. On such occasions he shows off his sophistication with a never-ending variety of quotes from great authors in literature and philosophy, which Lara clearly finds impressive. She finds learned aphorisms on her car, in her mailbox, on the door to her office. But also other frankly physical words about love, and telephone messages that go far beyond what a gentleman says to a lady. Never before has a man courted her so long and so persistently.

Is this the man who can satisfy her yearning? A yearning she has felt since childhood. She says she grew up with fairy tales and was always swept away by the great love stories of princes and princesses. Is he a Zhivago - warm, generous, compassionate, a poet and a healer? More and more insistently this tall, handsome man swears his love for her. There comes a time when she cannot resist his allure anymore. Lara takes the plunge, opens herself and becomes besotted with him, forgetting the world around her. Now only he is there.

But soon it becomes clear: he is no Yuri Zhivago. In fact he bears more of a resemblance to Victor Komarovski, the dark figure from Pasternak's novel for whom love is a game of power and dominance. Victor is a hunter who stalks an animal until he has slayed it. But before that he plays with his prey. He baits it, teases it, stimulates it. She likes this and doesn't feel a need to defend herself. All of her energy flows to him. At the beginning he activates her. It is like phosphorus: ignite it and let it burn. Like fireworks. She is burning for more. It is like an addiction. He takes all of her and she burns out. Becomes less and less. Physically and emotionally. She has less and less fuel to offer. Everything she has, she gives to him. There is hardly anything left for her other life. She is totally absorbed in his world, oblivious to all else.

He is her shell; she fills him with everything she would otherwise give to her children, her students, her friends, her familiar surroundings. She can no longer refuel like she used to. Cannot recharge by withdrawing, letting the telephone ring, reading or watching a detective show and later going out and tackling her work again. She gives up her refuges, exposes herself to him, even when she could use a break. If she is not with him, she is incapable of doing anything.

"A relationship," she will later say, "is something that always leads me to the brink. First I see the sunny side because I think, 'Now it's the right one'. Then I become blinded and play along. But the moment I open up, the destruction begins."

With Victor it takes months for her to realize, "Here we go again." She knows this game, she knows how it goes. And still she plays her part and submits herself. She doesn't just give of herself, she gives herself up. Hardly anyone knows this side of her. The strong, smart, self-confident Lara suddenly appears weak, dumb and dependent. She can't utter a complete sentence anymore, she stammers, asks for forgiveness for what he has done. She hates herself for this, but somehow she seems to need it. So she allows herself to be humiliated and feels like a dirty doormat. She does everything for him, plays the housemaid, cleans, irons, cooks – things she has long given up doing at home. She lets him reproach her, put her down, is obliging towards him. Next to her stands her other self and says, "Look, you need that now." She hears the inner voice but is no longer capable of reacting differently. She cannot turn the tables or change the rules of the game. Every time it ends with the loss of her dignity.

"He was the curse of her life," writes Pasternak about Victor. "She hated him, her thoughts stayed on the same track day after day. She was his prisoner. How did he succeed in making her his slave? What kind of power forced her to submit to him and surrender herself to him again and again?"

And he has Zhivago say to Lara, "Human nature, especially female, is so dark and full of contradictions! With a tiny piece of your repulsion you are perhaps more dependent on him than on any person whom you love! Freely love – without any compulsion."

Sometimes Lara stops at the end of a street near Victor's apartment, hesitates, hears this voice: Do not go there again! And then she does after all; she drives there and everything repeats itself. Only for him does she play the woman who has long since fallen apart in her old world. Her last energy is reserved for him. Outside of this, nothing functions anymore. She has given up everything that was once important to her, cast it aside like worthless junk. Work, friends, hobbies and last of all, the children. In the beginning he was friendly to the children, took an interest in them and even won them over. Now he has no interest in them anymore, and here too she is on his side. Against her own children. Ultimately she wants to give up her apartment for him, the home she has made for herself for over twenty years.

When he doesn't want her to move in with him after all, she almost literally crawls to him – like a hungry, begging mongrel. He should take her in, she will forego everything that makes her herself. He tests her. With totally trivial questions, with trifles, with irrational decisions, he tests how far she is willing to go towards self-abasement. When he lets up, she drives the game on again, a game that no longer has anything to do with love, and throws in the last stakes she has. She is like a junkie who hardly finds anyplace left to inject the needle. The inner voice has almost become silent. She is at the lowest point of her life, cannot keep any food in her stomach, can hardly sleep. In addition, she has excruciating stomach cramps and unbearable headaches. Her nerves are shot. Her children are forced to watch helplessly as she stares out of the window and no longer reacts. Her friends hardly recognize her anymore. "You're not yourself!" They beseech her to end this relationship which is destroying her. But she can't. She is incapable of moving or taking action, paralyzed "as if by a poisonous sting." Thoughts of suicide are unnecessary. She doesn't need to do it herself. The relationship with this man will burn her out until nothing is left of her. She knows it.

It is her children who finally convince Lara to go to the doctor. At first the focus is on the headaches and stomach cramps, complaints which are not new for her or her doctor. She has had these before in stress situations. But this time it is different. The homeopathic remedies she has been given in the past do not help as well as usual. And Lara is different: unsure, shaky, weak. The already slender woman has lost even more weight, has dark rings under her eyes and virtually no will to survive. Little by little she begins to talk about her other problems – her insomnia, lack of energy and drive, her feeling of helplessness and inner emptiness: "Between me and life there is a transparent veil." The typical picture of a depression.

At some point she overcomes her shame and talks about Victor. She knows why she is not well and still does not want to give up the relationship. She tells her doctor, "I am not important anymore, except in connection with him."

After Lara has been on sick leave from work for over a month and has been given various homeopathic remedies without any great success, she is advised to begin taking an antidepressant to treat her serious psychological condition and her insomnia. She is so horrified by the side-effects of the psychotropic medication, however, that she implores her doctor to try homeopathy again.

"I feel as helpless as a ship in a storm and have no control over my life anymore. I wish I could put my life in someone else's hands." This is Lara's appeal to the doctor. She needs an impetus to rouse her out of her delusion and lead her back to life.

This impulse now comes from a new homeopathic remedy. Five globules of this remedy aggravate Lara's condition dramatically at first. She feels as though the medicine is drawing together the last remains of her energy in order to drive out her fatal need for the game. It reminds her of labor pains. The painful release of Victor takes many weeks. At the same time, the veil between Lara and reality is slowly tearing open. She now sees her own role in this affair very clearly and is beginning to understand how it was able to come about.

It has to do with her womanhood. Her role models for femininity and love couldn't be more contradictory. On the one side there are three strong women in her childhood: her mother and both of her grandmothers. Women who work, are financially independent, who raise their children and are equal partners in their relationships with men. Women who know what they want. Mama, who died early, and the grandmothers gave Lara a big pot of love, a kind of basic feeling of security which Lara later seeks again and again. And they exemplified through their lives that weakness and defeat have nothing to do with the female gender.

On the other side are the women who raise the six-year-old girl after the death of her mother. These women submit to men, demand nothing, tolerate everything. Today Lara abhors the victim role that shaped the second phase of her childhood. She remembers how she was not allowed to express her own needs anymore back then. The young girl always had to ask how she should behave in order to be loved.

She had to be diplomatic when her choleric father threw his fits and be submissive whenever he beat her and hit her on her bad ear, which is now nearly deaf. Don't deny a man what he wants – that was the motto of her father's second wife. In front of Lara, she stroked her husband's penis whenever he commanded it. The man beat his daughter until she was sixteen. Today Lara believes that the blows were also intended for her mother, since he had never been a match for her strength and energy. He never forgave this strong woman for dying. For leaving him behind to stand on his own two feet with two small children. He never got over this loss, not so much because of love but because of his dependence. Lara's mother, the upper-middle-class woman from a reputable family, had the money and managed everything. The uneducated child of migrant workers, he received room and board from her. "She adopted him," says Lara today.

In her relationships, Lara copies her mother. She sees it as her duty in life to coach men. And love? For her it is something like porridge, something that can be eaten up or refilled. Lara gives all of her men, as she puts it, a pot full of love to eat again and again. She is responsible for refilling it. In her marriage she also follows her mother's example. A middle-class, well-educated woman, she marries a worker's son, who she manages and organizes. The pot of love is too big for him. The marriage fails. The pattern remains. Until Victor the glutton appears and Lara cannot feed him enough. She gives everything until nothing more is left. No porridge, no love, no Lara.

"In this relationship," Lara recognizes later, "everything which had been driving me towards the brink throughout my life came together."

Lara takes the medicine three times over a period of two months. As it takes effect, her vitality blossoms. She sleeps like a baby and eats regularly again, slowly gaining weight back. The pains in her stomach and head diminish. Lara has her feet on the ground again and is returning step by step to her life, her children, her friends. She takes responsibility for daily tasks and finally returns to her job. It takes three months for her to gather enough strength and courage for the biggest step, for her decision to leave Victor for good. At first she was waiting for him to take the spell off of her.

Just when she is no longer willing to wait, when she is ready to take action herself, she receives a fax from Victor. She can hardly believe her eyes. It says, "You must let me go again." The prey should let the hunter go! Then she reads confessions that would have been unthinkable before. "I know I have treated you unfairly sometimes." Between admissions of guilt he makes various attempts to save face. But still, Lara has the termination of the contract, sealed with his signature, in her hand.

Lara drives one last time to his apartment. He is already expecting her; he knows that she will come. They talk with each other for a while in a way they were not able to before. She is composed and her head is clear. This time she brings it to an end. A feeling of closeness is there at the end, like at the very beginning. There is a feeling of familiarity, a sense of what might have been possible despite everything. But then he breaks off, says nothing more, goes to the bookshelf and takes out her books, gathers her things together: vacation souvenirs, clothes, cosmetics. He deletes the nude photos on his computer as she watches. Lara goes through the apartment one more time, cries a few tears, bids farewell to the place and the man. Three streets away she stops her car and breathes deeply. She never has to go there again. How often did she stop here on her way to him, to gather strength to turn around? This time she has put it behind her. Victor did not defeat her.

One year later she will say, "I have conquered a lifelong depression. I am now the woman I always wanted to be." She has not stopped yearning for the love of a Zhivago, but the line between yearning and delusion has remained clearly drawn for her since Victor.

Commentary

The impulse which was to free Lara from the self-destruction of her love delusion came from *Cypraea eglantina*, the ground and potentized glantine cowrie not known as 'porcelain snail' in English.

What does the eglantine cowrie have to do with Lara? It is not its similarity to the vulva, nor its connection to the love goddess Aphrodite, nor its use in enhancing fertility which qualifies Cypraea eglantina as the homeopathic remedy in this particular case of lovesickness. "To cure mildly, rapidly, certainly and permanently, choose, in every case of disease, a medicine which can itself produce an affection similar to that sought to be cured" is how Samuel Hahnemann summarized the essence of his medical approach in one sentence. What kind of suffering can this homeopathically potentized shellfish produce?

A "blind date" was to answer this question in 1997. Without knowing what substance it was, 17 women and 2 men, all homeopaths, took *Cypraea eglantina* 30 C and recorded in the following weeks any noticeable changes in their condition. Every test person, or prover, was looked after and monitored by a personal supervisor, who also knew nothing about the substance being tested in this remedy proving. In this way, test leader Anne Schadde collected a total of 565 symptoms, with 228 of these in the emotional realm.

The symptoms of homeopathic remedy provings usually reveal certain focal points, organs which are especially affected, or characteristic sensations on the physical and emotional levels. The feeling of hunger changed conspicuously often after *Cypraea eglantina*, for example. A large number of provers complained that they had no appetite, as in Lara's case a frequent physical symptom of depression. Many suffered low moods after taking the test remedy. However, *Cypraea* also triggered other psychological changes which are very reminiscent of Lara's condition.

Many provers felt an especially strong desire for closeness, affection and love after taking the globules. They noted in their diaries: "Romantic yearning with very great expectations as of a fairy-tale prince."; "I feel like a budding rose. Wish for romantic, deep love."; "Strong yearning to really fall in love again."; "Strong need for physical closeness."; "I just wanted to be near him, bury my face under his chin, so it would be nice and dark and no one could see me. I would love to have crawled inside of him."

Such feelings changed provers' perspective on reality and they felt as if they were "in another world," "on another level," "far away from reality," "in a completely different dimension," or even as if "on a strange planet." One prover felt something very similar to Lara: "I feel inebriated, I feel like I'm walking on clouds, would love to stay in my world and live this ecstasy." This changed state of consciousness then had the same consequences as for Lara: "I am incapable of doing anything and cannot deal with reality anymore. There is a great distance between reality and fantasy."

The similarity to Lara's inner state extends to the choice of words. Here are some examples of Lara's description of her condition as compared with journal entries of various participants in the remedy proving:

Lara: "Between me and life there is a transparent veil."
Prover: "I feel as though everything were behind opaque glass."
Lara: "I feel like a lost, abandoned child."
Prover: "I feel defenseless, as if I have a very thin skin, open to everything; am weak, like a child looking for protection."
Lara: " I feel as helpless as a ship in a storm and have no control over my life anymore. I wish I could put my life in someone else's hands."
Prover: "I am helpless like a small child, I need clear guidelines because I don't know anything and I am thankful for praise, comfort and recognition."
Lara: "Everything is tumbling around. I am afraid of losing control. I have the feeling I am going crazy and am going to land in the nuthouse."
Prover: "I have the feeling that I am about to lose my mind. It is like a feeling of floating out of reality, without direction; everything is somehow excessive."

There is a clear similarity between Lara's disease picture and the psychological state which several provers entered after taking *Cypraea* 30 C. Thus it seems obvious to prescribe Cowrie homeopathically, in other words as a remedy which can produce symptoms similar to Lara's. Nevertheless this prescription was possible only because of a stroke of luck: the remedy proving of the porcelain snail was first published in the year in which Lara lost contact with reality. And when she begged her homeopathic doctor to try a new homeopathic remedy, he had just heard about this remedy for the first time.

In conventional homeopathic practice, a remedy for a case is usually found by checking the entries of certain symptoms in repertories, as explained previously. However, even in the present era of information technology, it can take some years for newly proved remedies to be included in these symptom listings. In Lara's case, a direct comparison had to be resorted to between the symptoms of the patient and those of the remedy provers. This was actually the classic procedure described and followed by Samuel Hahnemann before the existence of aids such as repertories or, most currently, electronic search programs. In the meantime, however, *Cypraea eglantina* can be found in the updates of the computer repertories under such symptoms as "lovesick," "confusion as if intoxicated," and "indifference towards duties." These new entries are based on the changes in condition experienced by the provers in the homeopathic experiment.

The results of this experiment are the first pieces of the puzzle picture of the eglantine cowrie as a remedy. They will be expanded upon little by little through clinical experience with patients who have been successfully treated with the potentized porcelain snail. The outlines of a remedy picture thus become more clearly recognizable over the course of several years. The complaints and conditions which develop into the striking characteristics of this picture are those for which *Cypraea eglantina* has been able to demonstrate its healing power repeatedly, in a range of people. Every single symptom of a remedy proving is treated initially as hypothetical; each one must then be verified in the therapeutic use of the new remedy. In this way, Lara's case was able to confirm some of the results of the experiment described above, as her state closely parallels the provers' experience.

Lara's case history has an additional significance for the homeopathic understanding of Cowrie, however. It places certain symptoms of the remedy proving, which were only momentary sensations, into the context of a biography, a destiny, offering us a more vivid picture of the remedy. Many more life stories like these are needed in order to understand the full scope of the porcelain snail.

5. The Land Beyond the Desert

In the deserts of the heart
Let the healing fountain start,
In the prison of his days
Teach the free man how to praise.

W. H. Auden (*In Memory of W. B. Yeats*)

It is a matter of life and death. Month after month. In the ovary, a follicle matures and the uterus builds a fresh bed of mucous membrane for the offspring. The hormone estrone prepares the woman for motherhood. Whether fertilization then takes place or not – the pregnancy is prepared for.

When there is absolutely no chance for new life anymore, this motherhood program is stopped. Everything connected with it is pushed out. For a few days the woman is left alone, totally occupied with herself. Yet while everything old bleeds and dies, hope stirs once again. When menstruation starts, a new cycle begins. During the days before, however, when the illusion of pregnancy is destroyed, the woman who was hoping to become a mother suffers. She suffers in her body and soul.

Sophia didn't worry about it for a long time. She didn't notice the abdominal pains and the very irregular cycle at all. There were more important things for her. Her married life with Manuel left no room for thinking about how she felt. For fifteen years she sacrificed herself for him. Since she had known him, he had suffered from severe depression. So Manuel was never the strong man Sophia had wished for. She had to be the strong one: caregiver, provider, therapist, all in one. She always had to cover for him, keep his condition hushed up and invent illnesses when he didn't feel up to working, protect him and coach him during his manic phases which were even worse than the depressive ones. Those were the times when he began working on a thousand projects, came up with absurd ideas, disappeared for days on end, then returned with a crazed look in his eyes, refused to take his medication and stood on the brink of the next even deeper fall into the black hole of depression.

One look at him was enough for Sophia to know what was to come. But when, when would Manuel take his life, as he threatened to do again and again? When she came home and the house was lit up and all of the doors stood open, she would see him before her, somewhere in one of the rooms, hanging from a ceiling beam. Every time she wondered if she would be able to do it without help – cut him down, determine that he was dead, make the necessary arrangements. No, there was no one she could have asked for help. It was solely her responsibility. For 15 years she had been mentally prepared to see him hanging, until she almost wished for it so the nightmare would come to an end. When she did find him somewhere, cowering in the depths of despair, she cried inside but outwardly showed strength and optimism. The worse he felt, the more upbeat she had to be. Until she finally reached the point where she said, "It's him or me."

It had never occurred to her in all the years with Manuel that she could leave him. She still remembers exactly how the thought first came to her, all of a sudden, while she was drying off a glass in the kitchen: "I can leave him. He is not my child. A mother cannot leave her child, but a wife can leave her husband." It was like a revelation.

When she leaves Manuel, no one understands this. She stands alone against her own family – her four brothers and her mother

– as well as her husband's family. Sophia's mother-in-law calls her a selfish bitch for being so thankless toward their noble family and leaving a severely ill, needy husband, to look for something better. The only person who understands Sophia is Manuel. From the psychiatric hospital, he writes her after several months a letter full of feeling and poetry. In one poem, he thanks her for having the courage to take the decisive step, inevitable not just for her, but also for him. It is like a blessing, an absolution which he grants her. Today she knows that she may have won her freedom and survived, but she lost something infinitely precious in Manuel.

For Sophia a time of searching for her own identity begins. Who is she without Manuel? But as intensely she searches, she cannot find herself. She knows nothing about her feelings, can't even say how she is doing. And no one asks her. Everyone only wants to know how Manuel is getting along. She feels a kind of anger about this. But what would she answer if someone asked her how she is managing? She would probably say something rational and explanatory, but nothing about her emotions. She doesn't feel herself.

Three years after separating from her husband, Sophia goes to a homeopathic physician. Her initial reason for doing so is PMS, her malaise during the days before her period. During these days, everything is more arduous; she feels sad, a sense of hurt and heaviness, and gets upset and starts arguments about little things. Since the separation she has increasingly noticed how stressed she is towards the end of her cycle. "Nothing dramatic," she explains to the homeopath, "but I don't feel well. Always the same problems and they're becoming worse." Every time, she feels like she is in a crisis. She touches only briefly on the difficult marriage with her manic-depressive husband. She couldn't take it anymore and therefore had to leave. Sometimes she sounds slightly angry and bitter because her own family left her in the lurch, with all of the problems she had with her sick husband. At the same time she regrets having gone too far in her self-denial and even having been proud of her immense efficiency. She tells many stories of excessive demands on her.

Sophia's voice is soft and full; it sounds steady, without any noticeable changes in pitch, often monotonous like a faraway magical chant. The soft, deep sound matches her appearance – refined and gentle, yet at the same time serious. The physician can feel how strongly she controls herself, yet Sophia cannot hide the deep sadness in her melancholy eyes. She sees the chance which is given to Sophia at the end of her cycle, for during these days she feels emotions, even when she cannot name them. So she asks Sophia to observe what happens during this time, when she feels more thin-skinned and sensitive, and keep a journal about her thoughts and feelings. For Sophia's silent but perceptible grief, the physician gives her *Natrium muriaticum* as the first remedy in the homeopathic treatment process, a proven remedy for cases of such deep sadness.

Sophia feels accepted and understood, even when this remedy first presents her with new problems. Immediately after taking it, she runs a high fever for five days, and develops sinusitis which makes her feel so miserable that she could die. At the follow-up appointment four weeks later, she still feels terrible; she feels suppressed and has no drive, but is still restless inside, and has sleepless nights with headaches and sweating. There is no energy, only a feeling of emptiness.

She says, "I don't feel myself. No vision, no dreams, no courage." This emotional state has taken hold of her since her separation. Now, since taking the remedy, she finds this state unbearable and overwhelming and describes her picture of it. Sophia says, "It is as if I were in a desert and I wish I could somehow reach the land beyond it."

When was the last time she really felt well, the homeopath wants to know.

"When I was a little girl, up until I was five or six, I felt secure in my happy, intact family, close to my parents and affectionately loved by my father. Then came the alcohol and then the other woman...," and here Sophia quietly begins to cry.

The day on which her happy childhood came to an end, on

which the little girl began life as a mother, is permanently etched in her memory: "We were five children – two brothers about my age, I was the second oldest, and the two small children, one a year old and the other not yet born. That was the situation the night of that terrible thunderstorm. It was a matter of life and death. I knew that. I could no longer be a child. In just a few seconds, I had to grow up, be a mother for my brothers and a partner for my mama. At six. I didn't cry. I was proud of myself and felt like I had achieved something. But I really didn't have a choice.

"Mama was desperate. I had never seen her like that before. The baby was due to arrive very soon. Outside there was a terrible storm which rocked our house. The wooden beams were creaking, windows were breaking. She carried the youngest child, who was barely a year old, on her arm. He was screaming. Mama was crying. She was in a panic - she was scared to death, I could see that. She screamed above the storm, 'You have to help me! Pray for me, Sophia.' There was total desperation and the awareness that I had to do something! It was like a mission. I took both of them in my arms, helped them into bed and covered them up. I comforted them.

"Over at the next farm, a light was burning. Father wasn't with us. He was with her. That woman. Like every evening. There was always one side and the other. The two sides were worlds apart. And I stood in the middle.

"A few days later, the contractions started. Mama knew that something was wrong - by the time the fifth child is on the way, you know these things. She had heavy bleeding, and the baby in her womb wasn't moving anymore. She begged him - I was standing next to her - in tears she begged him: 'Please, please don't go today and if you have to go, then come back right away - please!'

"And he went to that woman. Of course he didn't come back. No one in our rural village had a car. There was no doctor, no midwife in the vicinity. It took forever for my uncle to come and drag my father out of that woman's bed to take Mama to the hospital. There they said the unborn child was dead. There was nothing they could do. And then the miracle. The little boy was alive when they took him out. Badly injured, with broken bones. Her fifth and last child. My youngest brother. I was the one who comforted her. I didn't cry."

Thirty years later, in the homeopath's office, Sophia cries and allows herself to feel the pain. She has come to trust this warmhearted woman, likes the way the woman talks with her, enjoys the time she is given. After several courses of psychotherapy, this is a whole new experience for Sophia. She has never been so honest. As the daughter of an alcoholic, one becomes cautious and timid, always trying to leave a certain impression, even if it means lying. She learned to put up a front for others – first her father, then her teacher and later the psychologist. Sometimes she noticed upon leaving a therapy session that she hadn't really told anything about herself again, and instead just put on a show. With the homeopath it is different. She doesn't need to lie to her, doesn't need to put up a front, doesn't need to do anything.

Although she reacted intensely to the treatment with *Natrium muriaticum*, Sophia is open to trying a new homeopathic remedy. The injury and need in her soul have become even more clearly perceptible and her homeopath chooses *Folliculinum*, a homeopathically potentized and thus highly diluted ovarian hormone known as estrone (a type of estrogen). This substance is produced by the follicle during the first half of the menstrual cycle while the ovum ripens, and it is an integral part of the natural process of becoming a mother. Sophia cannot connect any positive memories with the follicle hormone. During her last encounter with it, she almost died.

It happened during intensive hormone treatments in preparation for in vitro fertilization. Her ovaries produced a surplus of follicles and the hormone flooded her organism until it broke down. Fluid accumulated in her entire body, flowed into the thoracic and abdominal cavities, her liver test values rose dramatically and finally her kidneys failed. Sophia doesn't remember details anymore. She only knows that she survived somehow. The in vitro fertilization was the desperate climax in her struggle for her relationship with Manuel. She absolutely wanted his child - he should continue living somehow. Yet his sperm cells lacked vitality. Here too she was prepared to assume responsibility. For life and death.

Sophia tolerates the homeopathically prepared form of *Folliculinum* better. Three months after taking it, she reports: "Things are moving forward, something is changing. My hearing, sensing and experiencing are becoming more acute. For the first time, I am having vivid dreams, wonderful ones and terrible ones. Before I was completely blocked and felt totally empty inside. Now I feel myself - I feel what is good and what is not good."

And something else happens. Sophia travels through time. Whenever she is driving alone, on the long journey to work or home again, during breaks, during quiet moments, her thoughts and feelings go back into the past and don't let go of her anymore. In stages, she relives her childhood. She looks at everything again very carefully, asks new questions and finds new answers.

"Strange things have started to happen, which I attribute to this homeopathic remedy. I started to wonder all of a sudden: 'Where is Mother and where is Father and who is who?' And: 'Who am I allowed to love and in what way?' There was a time after this remedy when I had difficulties with my mother. I really hated her some days. When I was with her, I almost couldn't stand it. She didn't do anything, nothing different from usual. When I heard myself talking, I realized that I sound like my mother. It was really sickening. The situation with my father too. I miss him terribly - I've never admitted to myself that I've missed him so much. Even when I can't maintain contact with him – it kills you.

"Back then, before it all began, he was affectionate towards us. He was an unbelievable romantic. He hugged us and told us how much he loved us. Mama wasn't able to do that. Yes, I seemed to be his princess, his only girl, when I was small, before things changed. There was the father who could be so affectionate and close, who loved us and was proud of us, and there was the mother who offered us security, reliability and continuity, everything we needed for daily life. Practical life, surviving – that was Mama; feelings were not so important for her. If we'd had only our father, we wouldn't have had a roof over our heads after two months. It was this extreme behavior of his, his passion that destroyed our childhood.

"For over the years, his secret, private affair became a scary, public one. Everyone knew about it. For my mother it was hell. But for my father it was also terribly hard, and today I believe that his excessive drinking began around then. My father was torn between his family - whom he surely loved dearly, his five children and his farming existence - and on the other side this woman who I now believe was his real true love. He lived with this conflict and hopelessness. The mercilessness of the culture of our region, the particular mentality of the people, their traditions and religion, and of course economic considerations would never have allowed him to make a change in his life.

"Our father was always gone in the evening. During the day he did his work. He built up an extensive marketing network for our agricultural products and travelled a lot. Whenever he came home, we peered anxiously into the car. We saw it in his face. One look at him was enough and we could tell whether it was schnapps, cognac, beer or red wine. Beer was simply disgusting, schnapps was terrible, but worst of all was the combination of white wine and schnapps. Then he was extremely aggressive. The psychological violence was often worse than the physical sort. But he was also physically violent. There were legal complaints against him – nights when he went wild and the neighbors or we children called the police. Our father tore the telephone off the wall. When the police arrived, he was like an angel. The same game, over and over again.

"The family dynamics which developed were dreadful. Everyone was afraid of a confrontation with our father, but we were more afraid for others than ourselves. We worried about our mother the most; we worried about her more than she worried about us. She was always the main target of his aggression. Whenever I walked past the kitchen door and our father was there with someone else, I didn't listen for a second to find out what was going on, but stormed right in and provoked him, so he would direct his aggression towards me.

"Over the years we all became programmed to direct the unpredictable anger of our father towards one of us instead. The boys didn't go to bed without weapons. One had a knife under his pillow and couldn't sleep without it. The other had carved himself a stick on which a chain was fastened. We couldn't take their protection away from them, but we made it clear that they should always aim for the legs, never the stomach. I also had a weapon in bed. There were times when I seriously contemplated killing my father. I would even have gone to prison for it, if it would have saved my brothers and my Mama. But it might have hurt them more to see me in prison than to continue suffering under my father.

"I developed an unbelievably responsible and close relationship towards my younger brothers – it wasn't really normal. Mama, who actually was and is tremendously strong, didn't show her feelings and my younger brothers and I couldn't sense them back then. I couldn't demand affection from my father anymore. And I didn't get it from her. It was as if the classic roles had been switched. For us, our father stood for closeness and affection. If you look at it like that, the mother's role was lost with our father, and the role I was given by my mother was a clear assignment: 'Sophia, you have to help me now.' I then took over both roles for the two little ones, the full responsibility and care and the emotional bond - all of the love and affection.

"I lost myself at some point. Maybe the day I broke my leg when I was skiing. The accident happened in the morning. It was my shin and it hurt terribly. My father was with that woman. Mama called there: 'Sophia has broken her leg and needs to go to the doctor.' He did come, but not until eight hours later. A broken leg wasn't important for him. Maybe I was testing him unconsciously: Will he take care of me? He didn't.

"For a half hour in the morning, I was allowed to be a child. It is my only, infinitely precious memory of affection from my mother. She wore slippers which made a certain sound; she came into the room where I slept with my two younger brothers, and woke us up very lovingly. She gently stroked our faces, then wrapped us tightly in our blankets again. She said, 'Six-thirty, time to get up.' Then she gave each of us, myself included, a bowl of warm milk pudding and we were allowed to cuddle in bed and enjoy our warm breakfast. In the afternoons, when we came home from school, she often stood at the stove crying and I wanted to know what was wrong. I couldn't do anything else, I had to ask her. Because I thought maybe I could do something and then she would feel better. She talked very openly and honestly to me. Always about terrible things. She dumped everything on us children, when she should have looked for an adult partner. But today she is proud that she never said anything to anyone outside of the family.

"When I was eighteen I thought I could never move out; I would never be able to get away from the misery at home as I couldn't leave the younger ones and Mama alone. But then I met Manuel, we got married and everything repeated itself. The first look into the car, a thousand times the same anxious question: 'How are you?' I probably made him sicker than he was. It wasn't the hard liquor like with my father, it was the medications that I could control, his sleep, everything. It's terrible but true - it was like I played God. I felt that I was responsible whether he lived or killed himself. And I saw it as an incredible success that I was able to keep him out of the lunatic asylum. I took personal credit for the fact that he never had to be admitted there. Yet that was one of the big mistakes that I made. That I never sought help for myself was the second big mistake. But I wasn't able to think of myself until I knew that I would survive if he killed himself. I couldn't cross that bridge for a long time. Later it turned out, though, that he could live without me. Just like my brothers and my mother.

"Now it is finally clear to me that I married a man who enabled me to live following the same behavior patterns as before. When I left my family for Manuel, I was leaving to live a better life. I had a good reason. I went to him because he needed me. His illness had advantages for me, even when I wasn't conscious of that fact. I didn't have to take responsibility for myself. I was able to hide behind this illness for fifteen years. When I left Manuel, I first realized how damned hard it is to live a good life. But I couldn't understand the feeling, couldn't name it and finally came up with a picture of it: I had been playing Monopoly all of my life. But I was only the banker, I never played the game. I knew the rules by heart. Now I had become a player and didn't know how to play. As a player, you have to fight for yourself.

"It was during that time that I met Andreas, my current partner. The question as to whether I really loved him was very difficult. His constant 'What would YOU like?' was something I first took as a rejection; then it made me feel angry. Andreas didn't go easy on me. I have never experienced anything like that with a man. He always asked what I wanted, not what others wanted or he himself. He continually demanded that I make my own decisions and made me confront myself.

"He said, 'I want you - I have myself already.' That was hard, really brutal. I felt as small as an ant. I was confused, without a vision or goal, and then sought therapeutic help. But at most, the therapies gave me nice ways of expressing things. 'You feel empty?' Okay then, empty! Until I found help through homeopathy. Beyond words. After the therapies, the emptiness only grew. It was a bottomless pit. Through homeopathy, I have the feeling that the pit finally has a bottom. Now it's up to me to fill it up.

"Homeopathy has made its presence felt in many areas of my life. My menstrual cycle is still irregular, but only by three or four days instead of three weeks. Right after taking the remedy, I slept a lot at the beginning. At some point that changed. I now have a lot more energy, a vitality that I have never known before. And resilience. I don't get sick often - the worst I've had is a slight cold. But above all I have courage. I have become more courageous overall. That is the central point which I can identify best. There have been wonderful moments. When I thought, 'I dared to do that' and afterwards I felt so good. Even if it was just something small: not thinking up an excuse, not saying 'I can't', but instead 'I don't want to'. Those are milestones for me.

"I can now keep a distance from my family. Until now I have always been there whenever they've called, whether they had problems with relationships or with the children or whatever. They didn't even have to say what it was – I was there already. Now I just don't play along anymore. Strangely I don't even have to say no or give some reason. I don't need to function automatically anymore. I can now take my place in life. And they have noticed that. They are learning to deal with this, and for me it is a little sad to see that it is not so terrible for them. They can get along without me after all. At the same time it's funny. Isn't it absolutely crazy? I sacrifice my life, my relationships, everything – and nothing changes for them when I stop doing it. They hardly notice.

"My motto used to be: My worth depends on being needed. I invested unconditional energy and endless time in my family and my profession, neglecting my own wishes. So much sacrifice, such a strong sense of duty. I lived past my own inner picture of myself. Now my partner is coming closer and becoming more important to me. Now that I know that I can trust in our relationship, I can be as hard on myself as he was at the beginning. I try to feel what is good for me and then do only that. For a long time that was very little. In the meantime we have started to renovate an old house together. It is wonderful there, like paradise. A dream is coming true; I always wished for such a house that can be a refuge for people who need peace and quiet for whatever reason, who are going through a crisis in life and need a way station.

"I still can't describe it, but I feel that I love Andreas. Sometimes I have doubts and wonder, 'Should I dare to live with this man?' It is totally different from what I had with Manuel. For a long time I asked myself, 'Is this love?' With Manuel it was an unbelievable bond, an insane one, what I thought was true love. Now I believe that Andreas and I love each other, but the bond is not as strong; we can also be without each other. My partner is not very welcome in my family. He is too honest. But of course he wants me and not them.

"Slowly I am starting to see the land beyond the desert. It is a land where I am a mother. A very simple, happy mother, with everything that goes along with motherhood - cooking, housework, play, and everything that I am, what lies deep inside of me. It will be a life, and I haven't felt this for very long yet, in which I play a role. A life that will take shape around me and not one which I will bend myself to fit."

Commentary

At first glance and from a conventional medical viewpoint, this is a case of premenstrual syndrome – a standard diagnosis for which there are various standard therapies in gynecological practice. For homeopathic treatment, however, the clinical diagnosis is of no particular importance. Here, instead, the focus is primarily on understanding the individual and their unique way of reacting. More important than disease diagnosis is the question: What kind of person is it who has this disease? The great Austrian homeopath Professor Mathias Dorcsi thus liked to call his specialty "the medical science of the person."

Thanks to this method of focusing on the person, Sophia's doctor does not concentrate solely on the hormonal deficit before menstruation. She looks for the context of this disturbance and quickly realizes that the PMS is actually an indication of much deeper suffering which urgently needs treatment. The doctor doesn't allow herself to be fooled by the symptoms which Sophia presents to her, which is precisely why her patient feels understood and accepted. Thus begins a process which is characteristic in the homeopathic treatment of chronic problems. "Beyond words," as

Sophia says, as she comes into contact with her past, remembers and questions the old pictures in a new way. After taking a remedy that works well, one indeed often feels as though a film were being played backwards. Old physical complaints resurface, as well as long-forgotten emotional impressions. Often first in dreams, then in daytime consciousness. And during the homeopathic treatment – we don't know how – the perspective changes and new answers are revealed.

Such a process of transformation must naturally be accompanied by therapeutic discourse. And of course many factors in the patient's life are involved in this process. Without the gentle yet steady pressure of her partner, Sophia might still not be able to think for herself. The potentized *Folliculinum* – she herself sees it this way – gave her the courage to do so.

As unusual as such a reaction to a remedy may appear, it is exactly what the homeopath expects of a remedy that is a good match; this reaction corresponds to the acting principle of homeopathy, as it was long ago postulated by Samuel Hahnemann. In his view, illness results when the vital force is thrown out of balance, and the healing action of a remedy must therefore be focused on this vital force.

This mysterious force – in Chinese medicine it is called Qi, in Indian tradition Prana – is as such neither visible nor measurable and therefore does not objectively exist, certainly not for scientific medicine. Subjectively, however, we can perceive it, and we can feel it as our energy; it makes itself apparent in our vitality and in our resistance to disease. It finds psychological expression in qualities such as joy and zest for life. In such terms, the first reaction to homeopathic treatment is often vaguely described. The patients report having more energy, better concentration or better emotional balance. With their newly found strength, they suddenly tackle things they had been putting off for a long time, make overdue decisions, are more active in daily life and have a new, more energetic outlook on life. It is as if their vitality were stimulated and more concentrated.

Sophia felt this effect as "more courage," but also as a new physical feeling and a better connection to herself. "I feel myself again" is a statement often heard in homeopathic practice. The story of Ellie's severe burns in the first chapter shows what a literal meaning this statement can sometimes also have.

Such a reaction only occurs, however, when the remedy fits not only the local disease symptoms of a patient, but also the entire person. With Sophia and her remedy *Folliculinum*, the homeopathic connection can be recognized in various ways on the physical and mental-emotional levels. The initial substance of the remedy, which Sophia took only once in the 200 C potency, is the hormone estrone, which the ripening follicle produces in the first half of the menstrual cycle before ovulation, and which plays an important role in the monthly physical preparation for motherhood.

The potentized follicle hormone proved very helpful in Sophia's case of premenstrual syndrome – almost the same as a standard gynecological therapy. In an English study conducted by Bruno Martinez, 28 out of 32 patients with PMS who received therapy with *Folliculinum* 9 C noted a significant improvement in their complaints. The homeopathic remedy had the strongest effect on bleeding, swelling of the breasts, irregular cycles and mood swings.

Yet in Sophia's case, a stronger existential connection exists on the physical level to *Folliculinum*, since she nearly died as a result of what is known as ovarian hyperstimulation syndrome. This disturbance is considered the greatest risk of in vitro fertilization. Because a sufficient number of ripe and healthy egg cells are needed for fertilization in the Petri dish, the ovaries are stimulated with the help of special hormones to allow several follicles to ripen at once. Sophia's organism was more than cooperative and produced over 100 follicles. Under the influence of hormones and substances acting on the vascular system from the overstimulated ovaries, the permeability of the blood vessels changed, fluid entered the tissues, the blood thickened and the kidneys were no longer adequately supplied with blood. In this situation, Sophia's life could be saved only through the most modern intensive medical intervention. As the trigger for this life-threatening condition, the follicle hormone had a negative effect on Sophia's constitution. From a homeopathic point of view, the substance can therefore positively influence this acquired weakness of the organism in its potentized form.

How does Folliculinum relate to Sophia's emotional state? What connection does this remedy have with her as a person? The British homeopath Melissa Assilem has used this remedy for many years in her practice and can therefore characterize more exactly the people who react most positively to it. She describes the typical "Folliculinum woman" thus: "She feels she is controlled by another. She is out of sorts with her rhythms. She is living out someone else's expectations. She loses her will. She overestimates her energy reserves. She is full of self-denial. She becomes a rescuer, addicted to rescuing people. She becomes drained. She has become a doormat. She has forgotten who she is. She has no individuality."

Sophia will easily recognize her old self in this description. Today she acts less on the expectations of others and more in accordance with her own needs. She is on her way to finding herself, her own rhythm and her individuality. Together with her partner and her homeopath, *Folliculinum* has accompanied her on her way, has helped her to focus her energy and thus given her the courage to stand up for herself.

6. Red and Blue

> *Wherefore, O judges, be of good cheer about death, and know this of a truth – that no evil can happen to a good man, either in life or after death. He and his are not neglected by the gods; nor has my own approaching end happened by mere chance. But I see clearly that to die and be released was better for me...*
>
> Plato: Apology

Sometimes Nora sees him sitting there, in his leather armchair at the window with the lace curtains, the dark red and violet plaid blanket on his knees, quietly looking out and barely moving – often for hours. But smiling. No longer in despair, with empty blue-green eyes under bushy white brows, as in the many years before. Now he was better, finally. There in that spot, the tall, imposing man seemed to be part of the furnishings in the tiny little house they shared. He was hardly noticeable, blending in with the doll's house, the voluminous period furniture, the Delft porcelain and hand-blown glass in the magnificent sideboard, the baroque pendulum clocks and the oil paintings on the walls. Nestled in his deep armchair, he seemed to have become one with the earthy carmine red of the already slightly worn leather. He said he was the happiest man in the world. Strange seeing so many shades of red from orange to purple around him, in the embroidered velvet pillows on his chair as well. Here they had finally stopped bothering him.

For the color red had triggered panic attacks in him in those terrible years during his worst and most violent episodes in the psychiatric clinic, when he saw the color in the paintings in his room, in the tiny drops of blood from an injured finger and then in the rose-printed dress worn by the visitor, that woman. Lysette, the other woman, his mistress. Fear, horrible fear had overtaken him when he saw the red she wore. Nora had therefore banned everything red from her wardrobe, even though she hardly wore anything this color, in order not to disturb her husband when she visited him in the clinic.

A habit which she kept after his death. Light blue was Nora's color; it was in her barrettes, in her long fringed skirt and even in her flat patent leather shoes. An unusually sweet light blue for a woman in her late sixties. But Nora is special, just as special as Pieter, her husband, though in a completely different way.

"Green," says Nora, "was Pieter's color." Perhaps Nora just sees one of the complementaries. Red and green are opposite to each other and still belong together, at least on the color wheel. But that is not important anymore since Pieter has died. And since Lysette (the woman who stood for the red in Pieter's life) no longer plays a role in Nora's life with Pieter. A few things have remained in her memory, for example that Pieter was happier than ever before in the last nine months before his death; and that he could walk with a smile past the large poster in the kitchen to the room where he slept with Nora. The poster which depicted a large, flaming red poppy in full bloom, like in the erotic paintings of the Mexican artist Frieda Kahlo, whose flowers look like the secret red blossoms of women.

When he stood up from his favorite chair at the window and crossed the room in three steps, he had to bend down in order to go through the doorway without hitting his head. He and Nora had often laughed about that. But they never wanted to give up their small house for another one. After ten years of marriage, they had both found the home they had dreamed of, at an affordable price, in a village not far from the sea. Nora could ride her bicycle to school, where she was a teacher, and they could both live comfortably on her salary. At 47 years of age, Pieter no longer needed to slave away as a mechanic, a job that had never suited him. His 34-year-old wife earned the income, and he stayed at home. Still unusual today, such a reversal of roles was certainly the exception in the early 1970's in a rural area with a very conservative religious population. But for the two of them it felt exactly right.

Pieter loved Nora because she was "pure," as they say in the Netherlands. Pieter was also pure or honest: he wanted her to provide for him, so that he could live his life the way he imagined it. He wanted to occupy himself primarily with contemplation, books and literature. In addition, he did the housework and cooked. Not, however, according to Nora's more sparing, health-conscious standards, but instead food that was rich and sweet, with the best ingredients and well seasoned. Pieter loved fine food, recipes from French and Mediterranean cuisine and above all, desserts. When they were first married, he baked a cake for Nora every other day, which was not good for her figure at all. So with strict self-discipline, she quickly backed off again from eating too many sweets. She remained slender and wiry, while Pieter's figure became more rounded and fuller as the years went by. This didn't bother Nora, and it actually made Pieter's deep baritone voice sound richer. His voice carried the others easily in the well-known *a capella* choir he sang in. Mainly Renaissance music, but also melodies from operas and operettas, folk songs and spirituals.

Pieter had grown up in the bustling city of Amsterdam, in a lively, liberal and socialist-influenced family, where topics were discussed openly and often. They talked about different religions or alternative lifestyles, and about love and sexuality. Physical love was for Pieter one of the most beautiful and pleasant things in life. For him, Logos and Eros played naturally together, whereas in Nora's house, principles and abstinence were preached. Sometimes he took Nora in his arms and called her "my little nun." In Nora's family there were certain subjects you just didn't talk about. People didn't talk much anyway, out in the flat countryside. Pieter, on the other hand, came from a lively community of orators and he soon became famous for this in the small village. He had something to say about every subject that came up. And the amazing thing was: people not only accepted the way he was, they even came to appreciate it.

Word quickly got around that the teacher's husband was different. With his long, white hair, he looked like a philosopher and he spoke like one. People went to him and listened to him like the ancient Greeks had visited Diogenes in his barrel. No one would have thought of calling him a sluggard or a know-it-all, for when he spoke with the neighbors about their family and work problems, he never talked down to them or over their heads, didn't demand too much of them and was able to accept other opinions. He possessed a broad knowledge of human nature and always knew what to say. He talked with them about what interested them, whether it was politics or literature, or raising children or dealing with insurance questions. He didn't keep what he read in his books to himself, but shared it with the whole village. Years later he could remember every word of an article in a magazine and talk about it in a lively and vivid way.

The visitors, and especially the female ones (for women were definitely in the majority) loved the afternoons and evenings with Pieter. Nora offered the cookies he had baked and was happy to have an open house. Pieter opened a bottle of red Burgundy and talked about how the world functions and how it is held together from the outside.

He often read poems aloud. Especially texts from his favorite writer, Gerrit Achterberg, one of the most distinguished poets of the Netherlands. Something about Achterberg's poetry and his biography struck a chord with Pieter, a kind of spiritual kinship. Achterberg suffered during his very short life from passionate love relationships and had to be hospitalized in a psychiatric institution several times. One of his poems, loosely translated, reads like this: "I cannot be born again. I jump about in the pain which is called giving birth. I am tied to a string as long as life. The most unusual and beautiful blue in my life is this Madonna blue. It makes me complete in this woman."

Nora was Pieter's blue Madonna, whom he worshipped and had tied to his destiny. But he didn't feel complete with her. He yearned for the red, the woman who stood for the color of passion and destruction in his life.

Lysette sang in the same choir as Pieter. She was 20 years younger than him. It wasn't to be a secret liason; Pieter didn't want to live a lie with Nora. Nora was brave. They lived in a ménage à trois, in accordance with Pieter's philosophy of tolerance and freedom. Lysette came to the tiny house to visit; they ate together, talked, went on outings together.

At the beginning, Lysette was friendly and thankful. Her life had become more meaningful through Pieter. Then she became a threat. For Nora, but also for him. She was not like Nora - not clever, not reasonable, not steadfast. She was complicated, impulsive and emotional. Pieter had the notion that highly rational people could live as a threesome in a totally natural way. But this was nothing more than a theory; in practice it was different. Everything went wrong. And Pieter was almost destroyed by it.

Nora tried to understand and they talked about it over and over, a thousand times. In the same open way he had talked about reversing roles in the early days, he now revealed to her that he had enough love for two or more women. This was a theory for men like Pieter, who tuned in to the Sixties' generation that talked of free love, tolerance and the good in people that made all rules and regulations superfluous. Why should you remain monogamous all your life? Why should you only be allowed to love one person, when there was such an abundance of possibilities? Wasn't everyone part of this abundance, this whole? For him this wasn't a theory. It was real; it felt satisfying and good. Nora <u>and</u> Lysette – that was his paradise.

It was so hard for Nora. After all, she was his wife. She provided for him. Loved him. She bit her tongue rather than throwing accusations at him. But he saw this and felt restricted. Lysette pressured him openly. She implored Pieter to choose her, now that they had finally found one another; she cried, begged, went into a rage. She needed him so. Without him she couldn't deal with life, without him she was unhappy. Nora suffered more in silence; she lost weight, withdrew. Lysette became hysterical, clung to Pieter like a drowning woman and in her hate screamed so loudly at Nora that all of the neighbors could hear.

Life as a threesome slowly became impossible. Nora considered leaving Pieter. As much as she loved him, she thought more and more often about living alone. Somehow she would manage without him. But Pieter would not. She knew that. And he knew it. Life without his Madonna would have been a nightmare for him. He was desperate and threatened to commit suicide. Nora stayed. Yet the thought of losing Lysette brought him to the brink as well. He would descend into one hell or the other, if he had to make a decision. The sumptuously laid table of life, with everything it offered a man, could no longer be. Both women claimed their territories. In the middle of the table was a dividing line. And so it went on: a cozy life at home with Nora, a secret life elsewhere with Lysette.

Nora continued to try and understand her husband. Why had he fallen in love with a woman who clung to him so? Why did he allow her dependence on him? It surely didn't give him the freedom he needed. She was the one who was strong and independent, who let him live the way he wanted to. Dependence and fear of loss were his problems. She knew that Pieter had grown up in the Jewish quarter of Amsterdam. In his youth he had witnessed the sudden disappearance of many of his friends, and his first marriage had ended traumatically. The fear of loss had remained with him. Nora sometimes found his fear a bit exaggerated when, for instance, she was out driving her car or when she came home a little later than usual. For him, separation meant being cut off from his foundation, from his provider, from life.

Nora says that her husband was "special." He could be sparklingly witty and was sometimes bursting with merriment. Usually he was reliable and stable - good old Pieter, a man she could trust completely. And then he could be anxious to the point of hypochondria, living in fear of death. Whenever he read something about a disease, he wondered whether he might have it himself. Only with a large dose of humor was Nora able to calm him down until the threat had left his mind. Then he seemed to be back to normal again, steady as a rock. Yet how quickly he could lose his balance. Until one day – Nora had sensed it and now had to witness it – he lost hold completely, and began descending, unstoppable, to the blackest depths of his soul, like a heavy boulder that tumbles down from a mountain peak into a chasm, until it comes to rest on the ground, smashed into pieces.

Pieter became ill. It seemed harmless at the start, like the soft sprinkling of gravel before the avalanche begins, and Nora didn't notice it right away. It was after his 63rd birthday and their 25th wedding anniversary. He didn't feel well; he felt weak. Then his stomach began to bleed even worse than it had after his separation from his first wife. A long bout of the flu followed, which kept him in bed for weeks and from which he barely recovered. After that came a painful prostate infection. Finally his soul became mortally ill. Pieter fell into a dark hole in which he was to stay for the next seven years. It was no doubt the medications, the many strong antibiotics Pieter had had to take for the stomach bleeding, the prostate problem and the severe flu. Nora had read in a magazine that such medications can cause depression. This gave her an explanation for Pieter's gloom and for his subsequent psychosis.

Back then she had to hide all of the kitchen knives, because he panicked when he saw them. In the night, shadows on the bedroom wall frightened him to death. Up until then Nora had no idea what a psychosis was like. Now she had to experience it with Pieter, who was literally driven crazy by everything. Even the most simple things. The idea that he could do the housework, prepare delicious meals, talk about his books or even receive visitors was absolutely unthinkable for now. He had become silent. Didn't want to see anyone anymore. Didn't sleep. Didn't eat. Didn't go out of the house. His soul sat in the trees and leered down at him. He was a heap of despair and hopeless confusion, saw ghosts, wanted to die. He feared for his life, for Nora's life, for the life of his parents. Waited every moment for the last judgement, which would punish him. The apocalypse would descend upon him.

On the dining table stood the rococo clock with the delicate dancing shepherdess and the quirky hedgehog mascot which sat on top, wearing a red and white checkered shirt. There was nothing to laugh about anymore. Not about these funny incongruities. And not about anything else anymore. The clock ticked. Only the sound of ticking carried from the living room into Nora's small office; nothing else could be heard. Pieter was silent. And suffered. There came a time when she couldn't bear it anymore and the doctor suggested admitting him to a psychiatric clinic. After he had pumped Pieter full of psychotropic medications and had already gone far above the recommended dosage, he didn't know what else to do. It was horrible. Pieter was no longer Pieter. The Pieter who Nora knew was dead. The Pieter she saw didn't recognize her anymore. There was no connection between them. They were two strangers in a strange world. His body sat in the living room, his senses had taken leave of him, and his great, warm soul was somewhere out in the universe. Nora was desperate.

Not another word about Lysette. Pieter had separated from her. In light of the uncontrollable trembling triggered by this visitor in the red dress, the clinic psychiatrist had urgently advised his patient to make a clean break with his mistress. Nora felt this was a bad time for such a decision. But it was made.

When Pieter was released from the psychiatric clinic nine months later, he was fully under the influence of strong medications. Staying in this state of vegetation was the only way he could function and ensure his physical survival. He remained a stranger to himself and to Nora. He lived and yet didn't live.

Three years after Pieter's affair with Lysette, Nora found another doctor, who referred Pieter to Dr. Sneevliet, a homeopathic colleague. Women were always more important for Pieter than men.

He found them more accessible, more tolerant, less dogmatic. Perhaps that was the reason why he could talk about his emotional suffering better with this female homeopath than with the psychiatrist in the clinic.

The first time he went to her, he was so dreadfully depressed that he couldn't say a single word. He simply sat there and looked out the window. She accepted this. Over the course of treatment he began to talk a little more, often in such a philosophical way that it was hard to understand what this all had to do with him. She listened to him with infinite and loving patience. Until she finally understood that Lysette was his heaven and Nora his earth. He described it to her back then in a picture: There are times when you come to an intersection. You can turn left or right, or continue straight on. But there are no signs telling you which way to go. You have to decide for yourself: Do I go left and follow my heart -unswerving, selfish, without a backward glance? Do I bear right and follow my conscience, sacrificing myself to protect another from pain? Or do I keep going straight on and die? He took the right turn. He denied himself the sweet, full and satisfying life he so loved.

Dr. Sneevliet tried gold and sulfur in homeopathic dosages for the obvious severe depression. These brought about slow progress. The psychotic episodes stopped and he was able to cope with daily life somewhat better. He became a little bit more the Pieter that Nora knew from before. But neither *Aurum* nor *Sulfur* were able to pull him completely out of his black hole. He continued to remain a mere shadow of his former self. And when they tried to discontinue the psychotropic medications, he immediately began to waver again. His stomach bled repeatedly and various pains plagued him. His fears still had a grip on him, and he was afraid they might put him back in the psychiatric clinic. And the yearning remained for the other, the one he could not talk about. He didn't mention Lysette anymore, yet he did meet her again sometimes, wrote her letters and talked to her on the telephone. Nora knew about it. Pieter led a double life which was not a whole life, neither with her nor with the other woman. In halves, he was stuck in misery. This went on for four more years.

Then suddenly his penis hurt when he urinated. Now nothing worked anymore. Sexual function had been impossible for a long time. How could he be a husband to his wife when he wasn't allowed to be a lover for his mistress anymore? His paradise of erotic love was lost and his penis had long failed him. And now he couldn't even eliminate his bodily fluids. They had to catheterize him again and again. This was difficult and painful, very painful. Pieter was in tears from the pain: and as a man he cried with shame as people worked on this most sensitive and guilt-ridden part of his body. The worst thing was the cystoscopy, which didn't work at first because the instrument was too short for his penis. With a longer cystoscope, they discovered a tiny cancerous growth in the bladder and cut it out. Further treatment or radiation therapy were not necessary; a few medications would suffice. The problem was taken care of.

Not for Pieter. Shortly after the operation and the painful humiliation of catheterization, he plunged to the same depths he had reached during the separation phase from Lysette. The worst fears, the depressions, the psychotic episodes, the fear of death and of God's punishment. He told Dr. Sneevliet about the horrible problems he had when they had to insert the catheter.

And suddenly the homeopathic puzzle showed a new picture. In the homeopath's mind everything fell into place, pointing to a remedy which would lead Pieter back to life and accompany him to his death. A truly worthy remedy for a philosopher: *Conium*, hemlock, the poison of Socrates. After the dose of *Conium*, something happened which Nora had been waiting for eight years. Pieter's soul returned to him. He became completely healthy again.

Nora had actually always known that the antibiotics were not to blame for Pieter's anguish. Yet it was easier for her to live with this version of the story. Lysette was something she had been given to cope with in life. Nora had been wounded, but wounds can heal and one can live with the scars. It was over. No, she admits to herself, it was not the heavy doses of strong medications; it was his sacrifice of his mistress, of Lysette in her summer dress, printed with red roses.

Now he waved to her when she stood on the ship on its way to Denmark, until she was merely a tiny point on the horizon. He watched the ship until the blood-red sun disappeared into the sea. And he was able to let go of her, finally. Nora was able to forgive without reservation, without the slightest grudge in her heart. Lysette, the other, was passée. He didn't need her anymore.

Pieter had finally come home. He was once again the man she knew and loved. And even more than that, a happy person who seemed to Nora to have been born into a new life. There was such a deep and intimate bond between them, with an honesty one can only dream of. They lived together with an openness not possible before, where everything could be said and done. With a love and devotion she thought only saints or enlightened beings could attain. Nora found this love with her husband and he could let go of everything with unbelievable ease. These were months which became etched in her memory, as if they were decades. She and Pieter. Completely reconciled. Without guilt, without regret. Pieter's being was healed. The hemlock, homeopathically diluted, had saved his and Nora's lives. Just as the pure hemlock had taken the life of Socrates.

She still carries these last months with Pieter like a treasure in her heart. His death also belonged to this precious trove. Pieter's emotional death during the years of depression and psychosis had seemed much more terrible to her than the actual death of his physical body. When Pieter became ill with an untreatable endocarditis and died a few weeks later, it was a relaxed and almost cheerful departure to another world. It was Nora who contacted Lysette and asked her to come to Pieter's deathbed, so she could say good-bye. She came, and they bade each other farewell without grief. Nora and Pieter parted with love, no longer together in life, but with the hope of being reunited in eternity. Pieter was able to pass away easily, accompanied by his family, his loved ones, friends and neighbors, so easily that the death of the teacher's husband, the death of the philosopher, became something mythical in their small village.

Nora made his gravestone herself out of clay. Her way of mourning him. The stone became as special as Pieter. On the outside, the cube made of ceramic plates appears sturdy, but in the middle is an opening, a cut-out in the shape of a horizontal figure eight, the symbol for infinity. For Nora, this represents part of her husband, the almost transcendental wisdom during the last year of his life. Precious time which will always remain a part of her.

When the green of the fern pattern on the stone was dry, she carried the heavy clay cube over to the cemetery and placed it in the middle of the plot. Every year on Pieter's birthday, she lays a big, deep-red poppy on it. Now the ninth flower since his death. His eightieth birthday. Next to it she places her most beautiful hand-blown wine glass on the light blue silk ribbon that she normally wears tied around her gray braid, and she fills the glass with purple burgundy. The clock on the church tower strikes eight. Nora smiles. And raises her glass to him.

Commentary

Of all the main figures from our true stories, Pieter is the only one we did not meet, with whom we could not speak personally. Through the eyes of his wife, we see him in a light that is romanticized through her love and his death. However, the perspective of Dr. Annette Sneevliet, his very experienced homeopathic physician, is also integrated into the narrative. She not only contributed medical facts but also focused on certain points which Nora would have preferred to avoid.

When Pieter came to Dr. Sneevliet for treatment, almost four years after his illness began, he showed signs of severe mental suffering in spite of high dosages of psychotropics: he sat there motionless, empty and silent. For this deep state of melancholy in association with great feelings of guilt, the physician first gave him *Aurum*, one of the main remedies in homeopathy for such a state.

Twelve years later Dr. Sneevliet says in retrospect, "For these psychological symptoms, I could think of a thousand remedies."

Indeed, the full-blown picture of depression displays few individual characteristics. Sluggish, spiritless, speechless; in a word, lifeless – such a state is quite typical for this illness in its worst form.

For the selection of a homeopathic remedy, however, the individuality, the indivisibility of the suffering is critical - the characteristics and symptoms which a sick person does not share with other patients diagnosed with the same illness. If we look at what is special about Pieter as a person, we quickly arrive at his tendency to philosophize, to enjoy life and not work too hard. We then just as quickly think of *Sulfur*, a remedy typically associated with this personality type in homeopathy. In the proving of this remedy by Samuel Hahnemann, in which a similar state of melancholy occurred in many test persons, we already find emotional symptoms such as "Great tendency to philosophical and religious fancies" or "The least bit of work is repugnant to him." In clinical use, Sulfur has proved especially beneficial for people who – like Pieter – tend to theorize and intellectualize, who are rather indifferent towards daily tasks and are hence likely to be considered lazy.

From a homeopathic point of view, there were therefore several good reasons for prescribing the *Sulfur* after the *Aurum*. And both remedies did help stabilize Pieter somewhat better than the psychotropic medications alone.

Pieter later received a series of other homeopathic remedies. Yet they did not bring about a real turnaround, a boost in his vitality, as would normally be expected with a well-matched remedy. In such cases, in which we do not progress any further, the organism sometimes helps us by producing new, clearer symptoms. It so happens that in mental illness, as shown from the experience of many generations of homeopaths, it is primarily the physical complaints which can lead us to a good simile.

This was also the case with Pieter. Here the new physical symptoms were displayed in the very area where he experienced such terrible psychological suffering and which was now mistreated with a catheter. The urinary retention, the problems with the catheter and the bladder cancer brought into view a remedy which had thus far never been seen in connection with the state of this patient. *Conium maculatum*, the poison hemlock, is regarded as an important remedy in homeopathy for tumorous growths of the glands and mucous membranes, and therefore also in bladder and prostate cancer. It is often indicated in urinary retention. And after *Arnica montana* (mountain arnica), it is the main remedy for "injury of the soft tissues," which is a general way of describing the complaints resulting from the bladder catheter. Although Pieter slid back into his black hole due to these problems, they turned out to be a stroke of luck for him, for the combination of these symptoms gave this experienced homeopath the signal for Conium.

However, it was not just the hemlock's connection with his genito-urinary symptoms that made it such an effective remedy for Pieter. Once her attention was drawn to Conium, Dr. Sneevliet quickly realized that of the many remedies that could be considered for depression, only this remedy addressed the core of Pieter's problem. What was this core? It was the loss of the sexual relationship with Lysette which had brought about this state of deep grief in Pieter. Not until Pieter's sexual organ was battered by a catheter and old wounds were reopened did this connection become clear. The sexual experience with Lysette was heaven for Pieter - this was why he fell so far after giving it up.

What does hemlock have to do with this? The particular effect of this plant on sexuality was already known in the Middle Ages. Back then it was valued in cloisters as a so-called anaphrodisiac, a proven substance for suppressing sexual desire. In accordance with the Law of Similars, *Conium* is thus used in homeopathy for complaints resulting from sexual suppression.

In 1900 the English homeopath J.H.Clarke wrote in his famous Materia Medica about the hemlock: "Unsatisfied sexual desire is one of the leading indications, and resulting illnesses in both genders are effectively improved with Conium." In the homeopathic repertories, we find Pieter's special form of depression in the entry "Sadness due to suppressed sexual arousal." Conium is the only remedy in this rubric and is also highlighted as an especially valuable one.

The experience of the old homeopaths is impressively confirmed by Pieter's story. Seldom has she seen such a deep-acting change brought about by a potentized remedy as in this case, says Annette Sneevliet today. After just one dose of Conium in high potency, he came out of his fixed state. Very soon he was able to drive, do the shopping, cook and be with other people. His fears had completely disappeared and he spoke for the first time about his feelings without theorizing. Most impressive, however, was the manner of his death. The happy emotional balance which took hold of him during the treatment with Conium carried him through the onset of untreatable heart disease to his death, leaving no more room for fears, guilt or delusions.

This is a very special story and yet in many ways it is not so unusual at all. It shows how difficult and long the path can be to find a really effective homeopathic remedy, how much patience and trust are needed for this and how strong the relationship between the physician and the patient must therefore be. It is also a good example of how deeply and lastingly a remedy works, when it addresses the core of the problem or its real cause. For this reason, the etiology, the study of the causal factors of a disease, plays at least as important a role in homeopathy as in conventional medicine. Hardly any other information leads as surely to a well-selected remedy as a clear cause, a recognizable trigger of the disease.

After the urinary tract symptoms in Pieter's case had directed the focus towards Conium and the suppression of his male sexuality was identified as the trigger of the entire disease process, it didn't worry the physician that the typical symptoms for which hemlock is known in homeopathy were not present. The word 'conium' comes from Konos, a cone or spinning top in Greek; as its name suggests, it is valued above all as an excellent remedy for dizziness (as well as for paralysis). These classic neurological symptoms of the hemlock were not present in Pieter, at least not in the physical sense. The paralysis afflicted his soul, his inner drive, his libido and love of life. Because the loss of an intense sexual relationship stood behind this paralysis, the potentized hemlock was to become an ideal antidepressant for Pieter.

The story of Lara was also about an unhappy love relationship which led to depression. However, she is a completely different person from our Dutch philosopher. And her fate is only similar to his when viewed superficially. For conventional psychiatric treatment with antidepressants, this makes little difference. In homeopathy, on the other hand, there is no standard medication for depression, just as there is no standard medication for any other mental or physical illness. Each individual patient is treated according to his characteristic symptoms, his biography, his peculiarities. And so it is not surprising that in our case histories, the four depressive patients Ruth, Lara, Sophia and Pieter each received their own personal remedy which corresponded to their individual states. *Ignatia*, *Cypraea* (the Cowrie), *Folliculinum* and *Conium* are thus only four of a thousand or more remedies which a homeopath may consider for depression.

7. The Lost Warrior

> *Vital to developing the homeopathic vision is the understanding of what is to be cured in disease. It is to be able to perceive, to feel and to know as the truth that disease is not something local but a disturbance of the whole being. It is to have the unshakable conviction that if we treat the disturbance at the centre, the local problems will be lessened.*
>
> Rajan Sankaran (The Spirit of Homoeopathy)

All or nothing. There was nothing in between, when Vijay Chopra tackled a project. A fixed budget, a deadline, the new factory. Ninety percent was not enough. "If everything isn't perfect, you've lost." He always managed it. That's why Vijay, who began at the bottom of the management hierarchy as a project leader, is now president of a giant pharmaceutical company in India.

He says, "I have made my world." Piece by piece, step by step, up to the top. To the very top. Everything around him also functions perfectly, just as he has engineered and planned it. His former bosses, his board of directors, his entire extended family – all of them trust him blindly: his reliability, his advice, his opinion. No matter what. If someone is in doubt about something, the answer is "Ask Vijay!" What he thinks and what he says, goes. This all-or-nothing attitude has become part of his flesh and blood.

"If everyone had done what I advised them to do," he says in retrospect, "none of them would be unhappy today." But some went and did what they wanted – the intractable ones. Why? He couldn't understand it back then. He was convinced that he knew what was best for everyone. Today he has doubts about this, for he now understands the power of destiny. To others he is still the same person he always was. The self-made man. The big boss. The general. They still see him in his full coat of armor. And how does he see himself?

"I feel like a lost warrior," he says now. "I am a lost warrior." He uses the word *I,* not *we,* as he did so often in the past. Wealthy, successful, physically fit, he is at the top, directing his company and managing his clan. No one has any idea that he feels defeated, like a fighter who has surrendered. "I wear a mask," says Vijay. A realization brought about by his illnesses, and their healing through homeopathy. Has Vijay lost his soul? Or is he now in the process of finding it?

His body taught him that not everything is possible. The last time was two years ago, in the year 2004. He wakes up one morning and cannot move. First he feels pain, then he realizes that he cannot turn his head. There is a terrible lead weight on his skull, which feels as though it weighs a ton. He cannot raise his arm, cannot bend his leg. Nothing reacts. He tries his fingers. In vain. He can't even hold the corner of his blanket with his thumb and middle finger. The whole right side of his body is totally paralyzed. Vijay lets himself fall out of bed. He doesn't scream, doesn't call for his wife. Using his left elbow and knee, he creeps forward. Like a dog that has been shot and wounded. Inch by inch. He reaches the living room, the telephone, the speed dial key with the private number of a friend who is a chief physician. It is five o'clock in the morning. The doctor says, "It's serious." He doesn't dare to transport him to the hospital in this condition. He is afraid of causing more damage if he moves the patient. Best to stay put. And take enough painkillers for a herd of buffalo. The pain doesn't diminish. Carefully they bring Vijay to a nursing home right around the corner.

There they are able to do something about the pain, but his right side remains paralyzed, without any control. After three seemingly endless days comes the computer tomography: a herniated disc between the fourth and fifth cervical vertebrae. The damned disc is attacking the spinal cord. This pressure, which he has felt previously but never taken seriously, is now so strong that it is crippling him. His nervous system is under fire: his sense of touch, his grip, his movement. Why doesn't anybody do anything? Luckily there is Dr. Joshipura, who has already helped him out of a hopeless situation once before. After checking the diagnosis, Dr. Joshipura recommends an immediate emergency operation in his clinic. The pressure on the nerves and spinal cord, he says, must urgently be removed.

Vijay begins to calculate quickly what percentage of probability would justify this emergency procedure. Dr. Joshipura is a very prominent surgeon and the president of the Indian Orthopedic Congress, which gives him points in Vijay's eyes. Moreover, he is a relative. Additional points for reliability. When Vijay was told he had terminal cancer nine years ago, it was Dr. Joshipura who thoroughly mistrusted the diagnosis. Vijay didn't die back then; he is still alive. These are all facts. Now this man is telling him to have an operation. Urgently. However, there is another fact: Statistically the success rates for spinal operations in India lie between 30 and 40 percent. Should he have his spine cut open, with a 60 to 70 percent chance of remaining paralyzed on the right side, perhaps even with further complications to deal with?

One can't be careful enough. After all, the tumor diagnosis was made by one of the best specialists in the country. When he presented with a high fever, Vijay was first treated for typhoid and then for malaria. The diagnoses changed, but the fever remained.

He spent 20 days in the hospital and the doctors still had no idea what the cause could be. They conducted many tests, came up with all kinds of ideas and puzzled over this and that. Finally they discovered that some liver counts were elevated and detected alpha fetoprotein, a sensitive marker for certain malignancies. Although nothing was visible in the CT scan, they suspected liver carcinoma. Life expectancy: 6 months! Vijay was just 42 years old at the time.

In his desperation, Vijay sought advice from his distant relative, who was very well informed about the most current developments in medical research. Dr. Joshipura studied the examination reports and did not consider the test results significant. "If you could base such a diagnosis on this, then my entire clinical experience would be for nothing," he said. "Don't believe this conclusion and don't undergo chemotherapy. Take a few weeks' vacation with your family and repeat the tests afterwards." Vijay gladly took his advice and went to a hotel in the mountains for a month. When he repeated the tests six weeks later, all were completely normal with the exception of one liver count.

Was this luck? Spontaneous healing? Were the diagnoses and tests all laboratory errors? Or were the conclusions of the specialists simply wrong? Who or what can you depend on, when confronted with the prospect of certain death? Vijay had decided back then to trust his relative and his assessment of the situation. And the problem had indeed vanished into thin air during his stay in the mountains. But he couldn't explain it to himself and when he later recounted this episode to the homeopathic physician Dr. Sankaran, the homeopath simply laughed and said, "I would have told you the same as Dr. Joshipura."

Dr. Sankaran and his credibility also scored high on Vijay's mental list. In 1998, three years after the supposed liver cancer, this doctor had rescued him in a similarly critical situation. Over the course of several weeks, Vijay had horrible episodes of abdominal pains and naturally consulted Bombay's top physicians for gastrointestinal disorders during that time. They gave him a large assortment of pain killers, antibiotics and antacids, with little effect. Everything under the sun, according to Vijay, was used for examinations: laboratory, ultrasound, color Doppler sonography, computer tomography, gastroscopy. No abnormalities. The spectrum of diagnoses ranged from stomach ulcer to intestinal tuberculosis. Even lead poisoning was considered, because the manager had taken ayurvedic medicines that can sometimes contain lead. The last expert wanted to give him medications for suspected tuberculosis. The uncertainty back then was almost worse for Vijay than the pain itself.

In this situation he consulted Dr. Sankaran, who was recommended to him as a top homeopath, and gave the physician an exact and organized list of the most important information. However, the homeopath seemed less interested in the facts than in the characteristics of the pain. He asked again and again, "What exactly was the pain like, Mr. Chopra? Tell me more about it!" Well, it was terrible, as if someone had grabbed his upper abdomen and pressed it together. This came and went in waves. It helped a little to stretch. Or to press his hands against his abdomen. When the pain overcame him and he broke out in a sweat, this was readily apparent. How often had his startled business partners asked him, "Is something wrong with you, Mr. Chopra?" Even though he hadn't complained. It was like an assault, so sudden and overpowering, and triggered a fear in him as if a bomb had exploded. Then he didn't know anymore who he was, lost his bearings. This made Vijay feel extremely shaky.

Dr. Sankaran conducted a two-hour interview with him and asked him some strange questions. Private and intimate topics were discussed, also dreams, and Vijay was certainly not someone who liked to reveal anything about his subconscious. But here Dr. Sankaran didn't let up. Vijay vividly remembers his constant demand: "Tell me more!" And he said more about himself than he really wanted to. He talked about his work and the all-or-nothing principle. Success and failure were always within an inch of each other. Even if everything worked 99 times and didn't work just once, it was all for nothing; there was no point in going on. "You're either 100 percent or nought." Zero. Nothing. Either you survive at the top or you're dead. In this situation he was naturally under constant stress and immense pressure. That was the nature of his job and it had its price.

High blood pressure and continuous treatment with beta-blockers were the result. And he became rather irritable, although he had previously been a very easygoing, even happy-go-lucky type of person. But this was changed by his work and even more by his marriage. He first became aware of this during his talk with Dr. Sankaran. It was his life with his wife Akhila which caused him to become aggressive, and at the same time introverted. His definition of rather irritable was: In the heavy traffic of Bombay, wanting to grab another driver by the collar and beat him up when he got in his way. It meant pacing back and forth in his office like a tiger and throwing a fit when someone didn't come to an appointment on time. Or getting angry when there was a grain of salt too much or too little in his food. He only went home reluctantly and could get extremely upset over trifles. It got worse and worse and sometimes he wondered what had become of his past joviality. But he just couldn't tolerate other people's mistakes.

The smoldering conflict with his wife gnawed at him and weakened him continually, for Akhila didn't fulfill their oral prenuptial agreement at all. He – smart, successful, in his early thirties – was an excellent catch. Regarded as a highly desirable son-in-law in the whole region. He could have had any girl. But he didn't look for the wealthiest or most beautiful; he had other priorities. It was most important that his future wife recognize the family hierarchy: his parents occupied the top position, followed by his siblings, his wife and then himself. Three of his five sisters and one younger brother could not provide for themselves yet and so lived with Vijay. It was his moral duty to support them financially. But Akhila couldn't bear life in a big family household, although it was only her agreement to this that had made her the wife of this wealthy and respected man. From her point of view, his parents, brothers and sisters all lived on top of each other in a house that was too small, where everyone could see and hear what the others were doing, and they constantly stole what little time she had with Vijay. So she made waves and caused trouble whenever she could.

Vijay's resentment and his aversion to this situation grew year by year. There were no verbal arguments with Akhila. It wasn't that he couldn't bear the sight of her anymore or even loathed her. He simply felt misunderstood and cheated. Didn't he give her everything a woman could wish for? Jewelry and expensive clothes, costly trips abroad, as many servants as she wanted. But her dissatisfaction poisoned the atmosphere. Of course, if he enjoyed his life, wasted his money on himself and neglected her, then he would be to blame. But this? He struggled so she could have what she needed, did everything that could be expected of a human being. Why wasn't she more considerate? She should think about what she could do to make him happy. When he saw that his parents and siblings were happy, that gave him pleasure; if he fulfilled his duties, then he was satisfied. He would love to have seen his wife really happy. He offered her all of his support, but over one issue was unyielding: he would never separate from his parents, never leave them or his siblings in the lurch.

Akhila protested quietly but conspicuously about her fate. Vijay became more and more depressed, lost interest in everything – neither television, cinema nor literature could hold his attention. When guests were invited, he couldn't wait until they left again. Nothing was fun for him anymore - he didn't go out, either to eat or to shop. The only thing that kept him busy and in relatively good spirits was his work. He spent 10 to 12 hours at the office and when he came home, he immediately withdrew to make business calls, or so he claimed. Because of his failing health, Vijay looked for a new job that would require less traveling. The new position moved him up even higher on the career ladder and his salary doubled. Step by step he moved ahead. Things in his marriage began to go better as well, as one sister after another left the house to marry, and Akhila had a baby, which calmed her down. It was a daughter.

Vijay had nothing against a girl. But he was absolutely sure that women in India hardly had a chance, whether they were illiterate or highly educated, poor or rich. For him, anyone who claimed the contrary was a hypocrite. The best proof for him was the misfortune of his five sisters, who were all attractive, well-educated and wealthy and whose husbands were in top positions. Therefore Vijay had decided: "If the first child is a daughter, then we'll stop there." After a son, a second child would have been fully acceptable. But now the risk of bringing two girls into the world and placing them at the mercy of this society was too great. Vijay didn't want another daughter - it was best for her that way. He wanted to protect her from the subtle injustice towards women which is prevalent in India. He wanted to prevent her having to experience this torture and himself having to witness it.

Akhila had to accept his dictum, although she longed for a second child and didn't care whether it was a boy or a girl. Yet when she brought this up, he simply asked her, "Are you happy with your own situation or with that of your sisters?" Akhila's honest answer was no, and so she had to go along with Vijay's family plan. But at some point she made a mistake with her contraception and became pregnant again. Vijay didn't think about an abortion right away, but "we thought about what we should do." He secretly had the gender of the child tested and learned that it was a boy. If it really was a boy and there was no mistake in the test, it was all right with him to raise another child. For his first daughter, he would spend his whole fortune and have her well educated, sparing no expense or effort to ensure that she got what she wanted. That was clear, perfectly natural. But he would only keep going if this was a son. However, he did not tell his wife that he knew about the sex of the child.

Since Akhila was already over 35, an amniocentesis was performed in the fifth month of pregnancy, to be on the safe side. The diagnosis, which was rechecked twice, was shocking: The child would be mentally and physically handicapped. In spite of this, Akhila seriously considered going ahead and having the baby. But Vijay appealed to her, "Your life will be an endless nightmare!" He still didn't tell her that it was a boy, even when the date for the abortion was set. Perhaps it was easier for her this way, since "we didn't want a second girl anyway." As they had feared, the abortion was butchery. The subject of children was now closed. Four years later, Akhila's uterus was removed due to gynecological complaints.

He became the director of the new company, his salary quintupled and he kept moving up the ladder. His little daughter Aparajita, which means "the undefeated", grew and to Vijay's astonishment was soon the apple of his eye, his support and his comfort. How wonderful it was to have someone happily waiting for him when he came home. When the tension had finally diminished, his father died. And a few months after this misfortune, he was overcome by the horrendous pains in his body and no doctor could help him. Dr. Sankaran had silently acknowledged the diagnosis of suspected tuberculosis and asked him about the nature of the pain on the physical as well as the emotional level, about his feelings and his dreams. "Tell me more." That was not particularly pleasant for Vijay. Nevertheless, he opened up to this doctor because he trusted in his excellent reputation.

After the two-hour case-taking, Dr. Sankaran promised that he could help. However, he didn't make any diagnosis and didn't reveal the name of the medicine. Vijay merely received a few white globules in a small paper envelope, and after three days his pain was completely gone. Unbelievable. It was like a miracle. He took the medicine a while longer; the pain did not recur. When he asked about the diagnosis and the medicine, Dr. Sankaran did not wish, as he put it, to go into details. Vijay only accepted this because he was feeling better and better and even noticed after a time that other things in his life were changing. He became friendlier, more easygoing and patient. And he was more willing to let others have their own opinions and to act against his advice. Colleagues and business partners saw how noticeably more tolerant he had become, and he heard them say, "Vijay, you're a completely different person."

Dr. Joshipura pokes his head into Vijay's hospital room. He wants to know if Vijay is agreeable to having an operation the next morning. But Vijay is not yet finished with his stocktaking. For two weeks he has lain in bed, semi-paralyzed, but he simply can't decide whether to go through with this risky procedure. He asks for another day to consider and requests a strong sleeping medication. As he dozes off, he remembers dreams from his childhood. He also told Dr. Sankaran about these. In one dream he saw himself lying dead, surrounded by his mourning family. It was the same feeling he had later when he came home from work. There he also felt as if he were dead. And there was another frequently recurring dream. Falling from a great height after being catapulted.

When Vijay wakes up the next morning, it is suddenly clear to him that all of his physical problems are connected with the deep shock he has felt since the death of his father. The abdominal pain that overcame him like an ambush in the months that followed, and now this paralysis almost seven years later. The shock is still there inside of him, as if it had all happened yesterday. What a strong personality his father had been; everyone should be like him. He was Vijay's sunshine. And he, Vijay, killed him.

Vijay is constantly aware of the presence of his father. From the time he was a small boy, he respected and loved him. Vijay's father was his mentor and influenced his entire development. As a highly regarded professor of literature, art and philosophy, he continued a long family tradition. The government had erected a statue in recognition of Vijay's grandfather, an important scholar of Sanskrit and classical music, and had even named a street after him. An uncle was a well-known poet; Vijay's older brother became a professor of English and Sanskrit and an authority on Vedic music.

Another brother is a priest. What a spiritual background! And they all had something in common: money didn't matter to them at all.

Vijay's father was an enthusiastic and gifted teacher. But like all the other men in the family, he completely neglected the financial side of life. Vijay suspects that thousands of students studied under him at no cost, for his only joy in life was teaching. He even gave the students money so that they could buy books. This drained the financial resources of the family, and Vijay had to earn all of the money for his college education himself, although this is normally the parents' responsibility in India. With low-paying jobs, he not only financed his own education, but that of his siblings as well. In this way he directly came to understand the necessity of money. It wasn't for personal financial ambitions. Money was an essential tool. If the others didn't see to it, then it was up to him. This task became his purpose in life. After all, it gave him the greatest satisfaction to support his family.

After he had successfully met the challenges during his college years, he strongly believed that he could achieve anything he strived for. If he really wanted something and worked hard for it, he would succeed at it. This was his deep conviction. And indeed he never failed. Until he made the mistake that cost his father's life. He still doesn't understand it today, "In my father's case, we lost all of our common sense." Even when he bought something as simple as a power drill, Vijay sought the advice of all the experts he could find. But when it came to his father's heart, he left the sunshine of his life in the hands of a single doctor, without seeking a second opinion. "We feel like we killed him." How often Vijay lies awake at night, reliving the situation, trying to comfort himself, telling himself that he thought he was doing what was best and the time had simply come for his father to die. But it is as though it were yesterday, everything still vivid in his mind. Vijay now knows how it is to be defeated. He has lost the most decisive battle in his life.

After his father's severe heart attack, the internist who treated him suggested expanding the five clogged coronary arteries immediately with wire meshes known as stents, in order to stabilize them internally. Today Vijay knows that this advice was absurd. When so many arteries are affected at the same time, the only alternative is a bypass operation. It wouldn't even have been necessary to consult a second cardiologist. One look on the Internet would have sufficed. But Vijay was so afraid for his father that he was out of balance, totally disoriented, as if he were enveloped in a black curtain. And that was why he let the doctor just go ahead with the procedure. The greedy catheter specialist even offered Vijay a deal under the table. Stents of the best quality, smuggled from America in carry-on baggage at a cheaper price than what the hospital charged. When his father's heart pain returned a few days after the procedure and his condition became critical, the internist suddenly abdicated his responsibility. A cardiosurgical resident stepped into the breach and discovered to his horror that a bypass operation had been necessary from the start. The catheter specialist had shamelessly sought to profit from this heart ailment. Vijay's father, who had blindly trusted his son's judgement, died shortly before a planned emergency operation, and Vijay was forced to look on helplessly.

His first impulse was to kill that quack. Yet this, of course, would not have absolved him of his own guilt. He knew: I have failed. I have killed my father. I am a criminal.

He had told his homeopathic physician about the death of his father and his guilt feelings. The homeopath advised him to practise *Dhyana* (yoga and meditation). In the past, Vijay had turned a deaf ear to such advice. But with Dr. Sankaran it was different. He had clearly proved his competence, his word carried weight and for Vijay he was almost like a guru. And although Vijay was not a religious person, he began listening to spiritual music whenever he could while driving to work. Ancient Hindu chants which soothed him and cooled him down. He didn't practise Dhyana regularly – perhaps once a month. And yet slowly his smile, which he had lost completely, returned and he began to see things in a different light. At the same time he experienced more and more often a sudden need to cry. An inexplicable emotion in his chest as if someone had given him bad news, and just as suddenly, a deep sense of sadness. When this happened, he took the medicine that Dr. Sankaran had prescribed, and after ten minutes he felt better.

Now seven years have passed since the death of his father, and the pain of it is still there inside of him. Is it this pain which is paralyzing him? Vijay has now made his decision. He has someone call Dr. Sankaran; the number is stored in his mobile phone. The physician comes immediately to the hospital. He says, "Don't be afraid, Mr. Chopra, and don't have the operation. Everything will be all right."

He gives him a homeopathic remedy, and two days later the feeling returns to Vijay's hand; he can hold the water pitcher again and adjust the bedsheet himself, and finally he can move completely normally again. Unbelievable once again. A second miracle. The rescue from an unimaginable misfortune: Vijay, patriarch and company head, paralyzed and confined to a wheelchair for life. It would have been horrible for everyone.

His daughter Aparajita, now seventeen years old, jumps for joy like a little girl, and Vijay would love to kiss Dr. Sankaran's feet. He now trusts him almost without reservation. Obviously the medical success with those terrible stomach pains was not just a coincidence, but a result of the homeopathic treatment. Indeed, it is wonderful: "We are completely cured." He does not have to undergo an operation with a questionable outcome. He will not remain paralyzed; on the contrary, he is as active as he ever was. Now Vijay consults Dr. Sankaran about everything concerning him and his loved ones. Colds, knee problems, but also illnesses in his family and his circle of friends. Always with 100 percent success. Dr. Sankaran can no longer be doubted. But Vijay is doubting himself more and more.

Even though others constantly tell him how much more easygoing, tolerant and empathetic he is now, he is not able to feel happy about this change himself. He has indeed learned that he cannot control everything. He allows others to make their own mistakes. If they don't want to listen to him, he is willing to leave everything to the almighty. It is their fate, their destiny. He even forgives

Aparajita, the apple of his eye, for wanting to decide things for herself. He has truly changed since the beginning of his homeopathic treatment. But behind his new equanimity, he does not feel an exalted sense of serenity, but rather the deep resignation of a vanquished warrior, the feeling of defeat that crept into his life when he married, that has controlled him since the death of his father and does not let go of him. On the outside, his world is as perfect as ever. Vijay is the undisputed leader of his company and his clan. He is credited with every success; when something goes wrong, other people are to blame. But he understands now that he is not really the commander. Nothing lies within his power. An inner voice, which is getting louder, tells him, "It's all just a trick. A facade. You are wearing a mask." No one knows this – only he himself.

Vijay is now often forced to think of his brother, the well-known preacher. How often has he said to Vijay, "You have to get off of your career merry-go-round. When you're 60 and look back on your life, you will complain, 'Oh, I've wasted my life!' On this path you will never reach your goal, never be free. You have to find out for yourself what brings you peace, happiness and comfort. Keep working at your job, but be aware that what you are striving for is illusory. When you're the general manager, you'll want to be vice president, and when you've reached that level, you'll want to be chairman. There's no end to it – even if you were the owner of your own company, you would think, 'I'm not Bill Gates, I haven't achieved everything.'"

Only now does Vijay really understand what his brother meant. His development since the death of his father is a kind of transformation process that can also happen to other managers. The old values don't count anymore. Money and success have lost their magical powers. Now he wonders what he can pass on to his daughter. Who here really knows what matters? What is it that is pounding inside of him, brewing, trying to break out of him? As long as Vijay sees himself as a lost warrior, he is still playing the old game. All or nothing. Yet he is close to a new awareness.

"Take off your armor, Mr. Chopra. Tell me more. Take another step. Trust me."

Commentary:

What a brilliant success story! Vijay was cured twice of severe physical disorders and saved from risky interventional treatments. The patient is infinitely grateful towards his physician and continues to place his full trust in him. Yet Dr. Sankaran is not satisfied with Vijay Chopra. Although the manager has outwardly recovered, he is stuck somewhere inside. He is still in the same place he was seven years ago, when he came to Dr. Sankaran shortly after the death of his father, complaining of unbearable abdominal pains. "I have killed my father," he said back then. He has been destroyed by this guilt; he believes he has ruined his life because of it.

No one was able to explain the violent pains back then. The leading physicians of Bombay were unable to make a reliable diagnosis, in spite of all of their technology. For Dr. Sankaran on the other hand, this was not a particularly difficult case. As a homeopath, he can treat effectively without an exact disease diagnosis when the totality of the symptoms on the physical, emotional and mental levels corresponds to the pattern of a homeopathic remedy. Vijay's complaints and his individual characteristics fulfilled this condition perfectly. His distinctive personality traits and his way of presenting himself pointed in a certain direction from the beginning. A man like him, a workaholic, performance-oriented, successful and assertive in the achievement of his goals, someone who always has to plan and organize everything, even the first visit to the homeopath, so that he does not lose control – a "Mr. 100 percent" like this is, from a homeopathic viewpoint, the perfect candidate for a remedy from the metal group. When he has also assumed responsibility for others throughout his life and has achieved a powerful leadership position, one thinks primarily of the heavy metals in the sixth row of the periodic table of the elements (see the Glossary). The best-known examples of this remedy group in homeopathy are platinum, gold, mercury and lead. In the life stories of people whose *simile* is in this group, we often encounter such themes as responsibility and power and their attainment, preservation or loss.

Yet a homeopathic remedy for Vijay Chopra cannot be selected solely on the basis of his general character. Like Pieter in the story "Red and Blue", Vijay's illness is preceded by a psychological trauma, which presents a valuable symptom as the cause, the triggering factor. In this case the death of his father marks the beginning of Vijay's ordeal. For the homeopathic analysis, however, the event itself is not as important as the individual's reaction to the trauma. Vijay does not simply react with grief or sorrow; he suffers mainly from extreme feelings of guilt. For an 'all or nothing' man, who does not allow himself even the tiniest mistake, this was his worst nightmare. Right at this most critical point, Vijay Chopra failed completely. His reaction is that he "reproaches himself" from the feeling that "he has neglected his duty", to use the language of the homeopathic repertories. This is characteristic for *Aurum*, homeopathically potentized gold. Yet Vijay's self-reproaches go further and intensify to reach the "delusion he has committed a crime". Under this entry in the repertories, there is another metal which lies very close to gold: *Plumbum metallicum* or lead. Alongside gold, lead is in another rubric which also corresponds to Vijay's emotional reaction to the death of his father: the feeling he has "unpardonably sinned away his day of grace," meaning he has lost all chance for God's forgiveness.

The choice between gold and lead was made on the basis of the physical complaints. The symptoms which *Plumbum metallicum* can cause in this area are known to us from toxicology, which is an important source of our homeopathic remedy knowledge of heavy metals and other poisonous substances. The picture of lead poisoning was already known in Hippocrates' time. Among the typical symptoms is the so-called lead colic: extremely violent, unbearable abdominal pains which come in waves and are relieved through pressure on the abdomen. Vijay's pains displayed the same character and the same relief through pressure, although he did not actually have lead poisoning; one of the gastroenterologists, who suspected this toxin based on the symptoms, was able to rule it out. The similarity with the poisoning picture, combined with Vijay's personality and his reaction to the traumatic experience, qualified *Plumbum metallicum* as the *simile* for the unexplained abdominal pains of this individual. The dosage of five globules of pure lead in the C 200 potency eliminated this physical problem permanently. At the same time, the irritability diminished and Vijay became more patient and easygoing.

And yet the feeling of guilt was like a thorn too deeply embedded to be removed along with his physical pain. It tormented him for many years until a new physical disturbance arose, more severe than the first. This time the problem, triggered by a herniation of the disc between the fourth and fifth cervical vertebrae, went to the very core. For the homeopath, everything indicated *Plumbum* again. Signs of paralysis, sensory disturbances and neurological pains are just as typical of poisoning with this heavy metal as the lead colic. And the backdrop to this illness, the unresolved trauma of "patricide", had not changed in the years since the first successful homeopathic treatment.

It is not at all unusual for different illnesses in a person's life to require the same remedy each time. Indeed, the approach of homeopathic treatment is based on the constitution of a person with its special way of reacting and its weaknesses in various areas. We have already seen with Ruth and her remedy *Ignatia* how a well-selected constitutional remedy can work as a cure-all in any circumstances. Drawing from this experience, some homeopaths believe there must be a single constitutional remedy for every person. Even though this idea is highly controversial, it seems to apply to Vijay. *Plumbum* brought about a second miracle for him, even more amazing than the first.

The fact that Dr. Sankaran is still not entirely satisfied with his success is due to the special understanding of disease and cure in homeopathy. Disease is not seen as a local problem in the intestines or in a spinal disc, but rather as the expression of a disturbance of the person as a whole, a "morbid derangement of the vital force," as Hahnemann put it. Rajan Sankaran speaks of a "central disturbance" as the root of local, peripheral disease symptoms. True healing must go to this root. It is therefore not enough for our homeopathic remedy to correspond to the local symptoms; it must address the core of the problem. And we expect that healing will take place from the center, that it will progress from the inside to the outside – as Constantin Hering already observed in numerous courses of treatment in the 19th century. According to Hering's rule, bronchial asthma, for example, should be cured before a skin rash disappears, and a patient should improve mentally before his physical symptoms subside completely.

Vijay does feel a psychological change as a result of the homeopathic treatment; he is more easygoing and tolerant and has more zest for life. He is no longer the old Vijay. Yet this is not wholly positive for him, for he no longer fits his traditional role. His job, the elixir for a workaholic, has suddenly grown stale and the armor of his perfectionism only protects and shines on the outside. An empty shell. The warrior has lost sight of the meaning of his existence. How can we evaluate this inner development? While the neurological symptoms of the ruptured disc have subsided completely, his psychological state shows the picture of a depression. According to the rule described above, this does not appear to be a positive development. However, Constantin Hering found that cure does not only progress from the inside to the outside, but also from the present to the past. Old problems disappear later than new symptoms. And that which heals last, according to Rajan Sankaran's experience with hundreds of patients, is the deeply rooted neurotic state of a person, the perceptional distortion that lies at the core of his or her individual reaction pattern. This dissipates very slowly and often long after the cure of physical symptoms.

In the course of this process, long-practised defense and compensation mechanisms can break down, with the result that people become truly conscious of their weakness and vulnerability for the first time. This is what is happening to Vijay Chopra, who now sees behind the mask of the successful manager to his true self, with his fallibility and fear of failure. For him this can be an important, albeit painful step towards inner healing. His self-image in this crisis still corresponds to the remedy picture of lead. The Dutch homeopath Jan Scholten exactly describes in his portrayal of this remedy Vijay's feeling of complacency, indifference and emptiness behind a mask, behind a facade which is maintained for the benefit of society. He recommends *Plumbum metallicum* for people who cannot give up power, although they have already lost it. There is thus a great deal which indicates that Vijay will continue to need his constitutional remedy. How often and how long he will have to take it and whether he will ever completely overcome his feelings of guilt is something we do not know. Sometimes his father asks him in his dreams, "Everything okay, Vijay?"

8. A Law Unto Himself

> *He who is slow to anger is better than the mighty, and he who rules his spirit than he who takes a city.*
>
> Proverbs 16:32

Wim smooths his whisky-colored wide-wale corduroy trousers and brushes over the black sleeves of his pullover. He sits ramrod straight. "Andy died on the road. An accident. Quarter past eight. In the morning. And on the same day my wife Lilian, a half hour before midnight. Cardiac arrest. No, no previous heart problems. The emotions..." Esther, Wim's second wife, picks up on his sentence. She is wearing a wool suit in a dark, warm rose tone and breaks into loud and merry laughter now and then during the interview. She asks, "Is it even possible to die from emotions?" Wim looks out of the window: "My brother also died from his emotions - that was why he died..."

In front of the large living room window of the small town house is a narrow veranda and a patch of green. Few plants. No flowers. The room is also plain. The couch on which Wim and Esther are seated is covered in a light-colored, cool leather. The remaining furniture is of smooth, light-brown beechwood, very tidy. Hardly any books, a few photos of children above the shelf, pinned to a board. An extensive CD collection. Classical and jazz. On the sideboard a miniature herd of carved wooden elephants. Esther brought them into the marriage. In front of the large, empty coffee table, a giant woolly dog. It also belongs to Esther. It brings life into the room.

"So there I was, alone."

"And your other two sons?"

"One is abroad. The other has a company."

"You loved the youngest the most?"

"Yes."

"I called Wim back then," says Esther and edges a bit closer to her husband. She read the death notice in the newspaper. His son and his wife both dead on the same day! That upset her. He must be terribly lonely, she thought. She was a widow herself. For weeks then they often had long talks on the telephone, and after the first date it was soon clear that they would marry. Christmas 1990. Twelve months after the accident. Marty and Tomas, Wim's oldest and middle sons, could not understand it. Unfortunately it led to a rift between the two men and their father. That was not nice for Wim back then. But you don't always have to mourn for seven years!

The relationship with Esther carried him through this difficult phase of life, in which he had to cope with further setbacks. His attempt to build up a small business of his own in his garage failed. Shortly before the new millenium, he went bankrupt because of it. Around this time the pressure under his ribs became noticeable - a feeling as though something were pushing together in his rib cage from two sides in the direction of his heart. He immediately thought of his blood pressure, which had caused him problems once before, eleven years ago. As was the case back then, his eyes were now also completely bloodshot. So he bought himself a blood pressure meter to find out exactly where he stood and sure enough, as he had suspected, his blood pressure was extremely high - up to 220/110. That could lead to a heart attack or something like that. His doctor said, "Your blood pressure is high!" Wim's answer: "Very interesting, I've already determined that myself." Esther laughs. The doctor, rather offended: "Stop treating yourself, that is our job." He prescribed beta blockers and they did the trick.

His blood pressure and heart rate dipped, but unfortunately so did Wim's entire condition. He felt terrible and he had no energy, either for normal daily life or for slightly strenuous activities such as bicycling. And he was depressed to a degree he had never known before. This couldn't be the right medicine for him. It did reduce his blood pressure, but it created new problems. It was surely this dependence on medications which made him so depressed.

Wim felt exactly the same way he had after the deaths of Lilian and Andy. Pressure from both sides, weak and depressed. It was the time when he had already started phoning Esther regularly and knew that they would stay together. Six months after the accident. Back then there were often quarrels with his sons. Tomas and his wife Cora attacked him from one side, and Marty from the other. Endless harangues from Cora. And in a situation where he was very sensitive, after all he had been through. They wanted something from him; he could feel it somehow, but what it was remained a mystery to him. They didn't make it plain. He couldn't figure it out – did they want money or something, or should he have gotten down on his knees for everything he had done in the past? He didn't know. They came, caused trouble, and left again. And it got worse after he told them, "I've met someone." They were horrified and asked, "What does that mean, do you want to get married, what do you mean by that?" And he said, "Yes, we're going to get married." There was a family conference and the result was their unanimous verdict: "Our father is a terrible person." Then eleven years of silence. Until Wim came under pressure again.

Looking for an alternative to his general practitioner, he consulted a specialist. The cardiologist also told him matter-of-factly, "You will have to take beta blockers for the rest of your life." And Wim answered, "Well, you can forget that." Esther laughs again. And the cardiologist replied, "Fine, it's your own risk – it's your life at stake." Wim retorted, "It's my life and I decide." The cardiologist held the door open for him: "Then I'm finished with you."
On the advice of an acquaintance, Wim went to a homeopath. First Wim presented him with the computer printouts of his blood

pressure levels. Taken daily for months, at the same time in the morning and in the afternoon. Meticulously and neatly drawn curves with entries for unusual circumstances, stress situations, weather conditions. Red for his excessively high readings, black for the normal levels. He continued to keep records during his homeopathic treatment in order to be helpful, and of course in order to see success or failure for himself. Wim didn't know much about homeopathy; he only knew that nothing could be proved. However, when he noticed how well-versed his homeopathic physician was in the sciences, he came to trust him. Dr. Scholten listened to Wim and he could see that his patient wasn't exactly cheerful. But he couldn't tell how terribly depressed this man was. Wim didn't talk about it. He spoke mainly about his work as an engineer.

Primarily about his invention. He was proud of it. It was the first electronic alarm system in a portable pocket design for heart patients and senior citizens needing urgent help in an emergency. You just had to push the SOS-button and medical assistance would come immediately. Before Wim's company could test and produce the device in the 80's, the small Dutch firm was bought out by a multinational corporation. His patent, albeit with weaknesses, was to be sold dirt cheap. That was not only unfair and unjust, it was intellectual thievery! Yet Wim could not find a way to protect his invention. He was supposed to work on perfecting the prototype for the new owners and organize the sales at the same time. And the people from the marketing department constantly interfered, even though they had no idea about engineering. Wim, on the other hand, had no talent for selling either his patent or himself. He failed at this task and then once again when he attempted to start his own business.

Calling something a production "weakness" instead of a "defect" - he was not willing to go along with such euphemisms. Bending the truth a little bit was not his thing. It was either positive or negative. There was nothing left to discuss. Wim was raised strictly and he was strict as well. Not only with his children. He was used to working hard and he had his principles. When he thought of the past and looked back - and he actually did this constantly - he had to admit that a lot had gone wrong in his family. Even before Andy's fatal accident happened and his wife died of grief. Back then he had been intending to work on their marriage, but Lilian's heart failure put an end to his resolution before he could fulfill it. Now it was too late. And when he thought of all that, it made him unhappy, even though eleven years had since passed.

How often had Esther told him that there was no sense in living in the past and constantly carrying this old baggage around. "You have to look ahead," she told him again and again. But it wasn't so easy. That was simply the way he was. Esther's words didn't help him. Even when she made it clear to him that no one could achieve 150 percent in all areas of life - work, profession, marriage and family. That didn't help him. People shouldn't point at him and claim that he hadn't done his best. Challenges were there to be met. If no one else was willing to jump in at the deep end, then it was up to him. Not because he wanted to be a hero, but because it had to be done. When you had to fight for a good cause, you didn't ask how and why. You picked up your weapon and went off. Like in Korea against the Communists. That was what he was used to. But at some point everything went wrong. In his profession, in his marriage, with the children. These were not weaknesses - they were failures, they were mistakes.

Wim's graphs (with the red and black curves on the calendar pages for 2000 to 2003) document the effect the prescribed remedies had on his blood pressure during homeopathic treatment. The changes in his emotions ran parallel. The first remedy was the oxide of the metalloid antimony, which was already described by the Roman chronicler Pliny as an "eye enlarger." With this, Wim's blood pressure went down, but only for three months. During this time something stirred in him. He felt emotions he wasn't used to, similar to when he was in the army in the tropics, when the malaria began. A kind of heaviness when he thought of his dead son or of his wrong reactions towards his wife. He also thought of his father. He became more conscious of the spoiled relationship between Marty, Tomas and himself and the devastating actions of his new bosses that drove him into a defensive position when he was normally the aggressor.

Esther pats the dog. Everyone sounds off about feelings. But there is no consensus about what a feeling is. The newest research findings on feelings seem plausible to Wim. They reduce everything to the two poles of attraction and repulsion, pleasant and unpleasant, positive and negative. But emotions are different from feelings. Emotions flow and swirl constantly inside of a person, often intangible and unconscious, often deeply hidden and scarcely discernible on the surface. Feelings are something conscious, things which become thoughts that can be expressed and shared.

After the globules, Wim's swirling emotions became feelings. He sometimes felt like an alien or as if he were in a time machine. It took him back to the 1950's, when he was newly married and was a professional soldier. And he felt the disappointment and the great sadness he had experienced in this earlier phase of his life. His dreams were like old films. Of his company, the army, his childhood when he was very small, frightened of the eerie things hiding under his bed. Now he saw himself in a dream on his way to roll call, but he was not dressed according to regulations and so he wouldn't be able to get there on time. The bosses of his old company and the new corporation appeared arm-in-arm in his nightmares and accused him of making mistakes in the design of his device. Even though he tried his best, he couldn't find the mistakes and make the thing work. And he fell again and again into unending blackness. He felt shame, humiliation, anger. And he was afraid.

"What was I like as a child?" Wim doesn't grin at all. "I was wild and always reacted to things very quickly. I was not a nice child." Here Esther laughs warmly again. Wim was a real roughneck, quick to use his fists, especially in the name of justice. If fight clubs had existed in his youth, he would have joined one.

"I needed a reaction to my action." But no, he wasn't a brainless daredevil, or even an impulsive type. He thought it over first before taking action. Yet he did not recoil from disputes and he had his own laws. He was not a criminal, but sometimes dangerously close. Here and there he tore a plank out of a fence or destroyed a bicycle, but he never wanted to hurt anyone. He just enjoyed playing with fire.

Once the fire got out of hand. Of course Esther knows this story. She knows what is coming; she is familiar with Wim's dry way of telling it. Well, he was roaming around in the woods with his gang and they made a little fire. Playing with matches somewhere was a popular way for the boys to pass the time. But the flames spread and soon the whole forest was ablaze. It was a real forest fire, and the local fire department took a long time to get it under control. His father was not one to lay a hand on his children, but he did so in this instance for the first time. And Esther just has to laugh again and again, for there is another funny story connected with the second time that Wim's father thrashed his son. And Wim tells it with a completely straight face. It was in the town on the coast where he lived for a while with his family, and his parents came back from shopping and saw a boy walking around up on the roof of a house. Wim's father saw this from a distance and said, "If that's who I think it is, he's going to get a thrashing." He caught his son at the back of the house. Wim was about eleven years old at the time.

One year later, his father died. Wim had already almost lost him once. At that time he was almost two and could already talk amazingly well. After his father had a serious car accident, Wim stopped talking and didn't start again until he was three. The death of his father changed the twelve-year-old in a similar way. He became more serious, quiet, contemplative. His mother hardly noticed. She had to provide for the children herself. There was no money. It was wartime. She often struck her son, even for small things, sometimes with the iron rod used for drying clothes at the oven, when she could get her hands on it. That was not fair. His father had only struck him twice in his whole life. Because of the forest fire and because of his walk on the roof. That was fair.

As a child, he already knew that he was not capable of being as perfect as he wanted to be. But he was ambitious. Poor at reading and writing due to dyslexia, he focused on technical subjects and mathematics. There he could show that he was the best. Not with his mouth, not with words. He wanted hard evidence, solid proof. Is he the best or not? And then if he succeeded: Look here, it's me!

When he was unjustly criticized or blamed, Wim could go crazy, but over time he thought more and more about the words of one of the few teachers who was there for him: "Whoever can conquer himself is stronger than someone who conquers an entire city." And because Wim wanted to learn that for himself and his future life, he enlisted in the military. It was his only chance. A notice in the newspaper advertised free college studies in the navy. It's the same the world over – the military paid the way for a young man who had nothing else. Wim served for ten years as a radio technician and soldier.

Wim spoke to his homeopathic physician more and more often about his childhood. He talked about the unfamiliar torrents of feelings, the dreams, the deep sadness he still felt about Andy's death; and he now talked openly about his depression. A buried side of his being had come to the surface like the inner layers of an onion. For this layer of his personality he received a different remedy: *Natrium carbonicum*, soda. And after a while he was able to let go of these gloomy thoughts connected with the past, let go of the compulsion to constantly look back and regret what had happened. He still wasn't optimistic about the future, however, and his blood pressure didn't stabilize over the long term.

Dr. Scholten questioned him more intensively regarding his feelings about the loss of his invention and the collapse of his old company. To Wim, the company had been "sucked dry" and laid waste. Being cheated out of his patent felt "as though someone had taken away my brainchild." Like Andy, his youngest child, a man after his own heart, more like Wim than his other sons. Although he was only 20, he was the first of the three to find a good job, whereas the others took a long time to find an occupation. And he was the only one who completed his military service. Tomas, the middle son, was deaf in one ear and thus unfit for service.

And Marty, who had long hair and played the piano day and night, was a pacifist. He regarded his father as an authoritarian fuddy-duddy who wanted to bend his son to fit his mold. Again and again Marty attacked Wim: "My dear father, you are so domineering. Do you want to bludgeon me into becoming an electrical technician?" He wanted to go to the Conservatory. Marty rebelled fiercely, whereas Tomas was taciturn. But both were in agreement: there's no way we want to be like our old man.

Wim had served in the Korean War out of conviction. He wanted to be brave and do his best for a good cause. Marty was against war, against the atomic bomb, against fighting and violence. Talk things over instead. Smoke dope and hang out, don't think about anything sensible, become a musician. Peace! But that was why he always took a beating. Wim had never been like that. He didn't wait until someone attacked him; he took action long before it got that far. He wanted to be the strongest. Better not to wait until you had your back to the wall.

Esther serves tea and cookies. The dog roams around the table, sits on command and wags his tail. Go outside? His eyes are begging.

"I was too strict and domineering with my children," says Wim. And Esther nods. Wim questions the tough principles he had back then: "What was true before may not be true today. They used to say: If you do good, you'll go to heaven, and if you're bad, you'll be off to hell! Yet the truth is…but what is the truth anyway? The truth is complex, it's something different for each person."

Dr. Scholten felt his way over the course of two years towards Wim's truth – or truths. During this time he gave his patient several remedies which helped further. A few globules of *Chenopodium* (a potentized plant called goosefoot) put paid to a chronic ear inflammation that Wim had suffered for years and that was resistant to antibiotics. His bi-monthly visits to a specialist for ear lavages were no longer necessary. Time and again, Wim was amazed at what these small globules could do. Actually he had an aversion towards doctors. They always thought they knew best. From Jan Scholten, on the other hand, he learned a lot about causes and symptoms and that a person cannot simply be repaired like a machine. That impressed him.

The real breakthrough then came with a remedy that was as yet completely unknown. Wim was one of the first patients to be treated with *Neodymium oxydatum*. With this therapy, he felt a tremendous pressure in his chest for a few days, and his blood pressure increased dramatically, before becoming completely normal again. For three years now the levels have been better than with the beta blockers; his accurate graphs leave no room for doubt about that. Wim presented them to his former general practitioner, taking pains not to gloat too openly. The doctor simply didn't believe this was possible without the conventional hypertension medications. Wim gave him Dr. Scholten's address and left.

What else has changed with this unpronounceable remedy?

Wim: "Well, first I wasn't as depressed anymore - now I could see things in a good light some days, though not every day."

Esther: "Before, you were always pessimistic."

Wim: "Afterwards I was able to look on the bright side of life."

Esther: "See, I always saw the bright side of life - I always told you to look ahead."

Wim: "Exactly. You always see the bright side, but there are two sides."

He remembers clearly the first weeks after the new remedy. This *Neodymium oxydatum* made him more than optimistic; he became almost carefree. Esther laughs loudly and warmly. "He went off with our camper, not knowing where he would end up. He didn't even check whether the fuel tank was full. And he didn't take the spare fuel container either. Before he used to check everything and think too much before doing something." As such incidents occurred more frequently, she began to wonder: "Is this another man?"

Now he is once again able to look before he leaps. He is balanced. He may not drive off without the spare fuel container anymore, but he can still say: "Let's go on a trip, sweetheart!" It is a totally new freedom. "Sweetheart!" Esther enjoys this very much. And he has more energy than ever before in his life. Although he is now over 70. He is always busy with something, making plans and looking forward to each new day. He calls his energy "concentration and calculable stabilization." On a scale from 0 to 100, it went from 30 to 50 with the first homeopathic remedies, then stayed for a long time at 60, and then with the *Neodymium* jumped up to 90. His quality of life has increased from an average of 40 to 90. Before he always had the feeling "I have to!" He needed pressure, a great deal of pressure. Now this has gone and he is much more easygoing.

"I feel stress-free and balanced," says Wim. His relationship with his sons is also improving slowly. Tomas has become closer to him again since his divorce from Cora. She went off with his neighbor. Wim tries hard not to smile at that. And oh, Marty called - the first time in 16 years. He wanted advice from his father. He has problems. Wim was unbelievably sensitive and careful on the telephone so as not to damage the tender shoots of a budding new relationship with his oldest son. Of course he looks back occasionally. "But I can live with it today - before, I couldn't." In retrospect he compares the experiences of the last few years to the peeling of an onion. One layer of his being after another came to the fore. He says, and here his tone is almost reverential: "I can now feel how I can continue to grow. Inside I have the feeling I can survive - I'm moving forward, I'm doing what I want to."

He holds his homeopathic physician in high regard for his knowledge and his humor, but it is ultimately the real proof of homeopathy's effectiveness that convinces him.

"I would never have believed that homeopathy would do this

with my whole body and ..." (here Wim takes a long pause and Esther is silent) "...my feelings." The dog has laid his snout on Wim's left knee. On Wim's right knee lies Esther's hand.

Commentary:

The main person in this story reminds us in many ways of the "lost warrior" in the last chapter. Like him, Wim arrives at the first consultation well prepared, with accurate records. He is also a perfectionist who must always check everything, who cannot allow himself to make mistakes and who is thus constantly under a great deal of pressure. His perspective on the world is clearly structured into categories of black and white, positive and negative. He hardly speaks about feelings; he is a man of action. The parallels with Vijay lead us to suspect that Wim needs a similar homeopathic remedy, a remedy from the realm of metals.

This approach (narrowing the selection of a homeopathic remedy to one or more groups of similar substances, on the basis of a patient's characteristic traits and symptoms) is called group analysis. It was Jan Scholten from Utrecht who was instrumental in developing this method of analysis in the 1990's. To be able to understand his method in Wim's case, we need to learn about his scientific work in more detail. Proceeding from the assumption that substances with similar physical and chemical properties must also be related in their homeopathic effect, the Dutch homeopath and chemist made the periodic table of the elements accessible for use in homeopathy (organising it slightly differently in some aspects).

Introduced to chemistry by Dmitri Mendeleev in the 19th century, the coordinate system shows in horizontal rows elements that are physically close to each other. Scholten searched for common characteristics of the substances used in homeopathy for each of the seven rows (known as periods). Almost half of the naturally occurring elements have long been used as homeopathic remedies. For the well-known remedy substances potassium, calcium, iron, copper, zinc and arsenic (which are all in the fourth row of the periodic table) Scholten found such common themes as work, duty, order, routine, rules. In the lives of people needing one of these remedies, these themes are often relevant. On the other hand, when the themes revolve around power and responsibility, as with Vijay Chopra, the Indian executive, we tend to think of homeopathic remedies from the sixth row of the periodic table.

With the help of the 18 vertical columns known as groups, the substances can be differentiated further. Just as the elements of a group react in a similar way chemically, Scholten also found a certain psycho-physical reaction type for the homeopathic remedies in the same group. Let's look at Vijay Chopra and his remedy, *Plumbum metallicum*. Lead (Pb) is in the 14th of the 18 groups in the periodic table (see the Glossary). Stannum or Tin (Sn) is the other element in Group 14 used in homeopathy. As a typical reaction pattern of people needing one of these remedies, Scholten found the compulsion to maintain formalities and to hide the loss of previous strength behind a perfect facade. Plumbum is from the sixth row of the periodic table, with its focus on power and responsibility; thus Vijay is concerned with keeping up the appearance of his old position of power, although he himself knows that he cannot fulfill this position, knows that it is now no more than an empty shell.

Scholten's work to define themes and patterns within the 18 groups (in columns) and 7 periods (in rows) opens up a realm of amazing possibilities. Mendeleev was able not only to predict the existence of a number of chemical elements unknown at that time, but also to derive many of their characteristics. In the same way, important traits of new homeopathic remedies from the natural realm can be postulated in accordance with Scholten's system. Consider, for example, Germanium (Ge), a metal from the fourth row of the periodic table which was discovered in 1886 in accordance with Mendeleev's predictions. Like lead and tin, this element is in Group 14. Using Scholten's system, if we cross the

Group 14 pattern with the Row 4 themes mentioned above, we obtain the picture of a person who is frozen in his order and routine, a civil servant who hides behind rules and regulations and whose real personality behind the mask of duty and bureaucracy cannot be discerned.

Of course such a character is initially nothing more than a hypothesis. In the twelve years since Jan Scholten publicized his main model with an entire series of extrapolated remedy pictures, numerous colleagues around the world have used these new remedies in practice, thus putting the system to the test. With therapeutic success, it has been possible to confirm the predictions in many cases. In this way, scientific development in homeopathy has reached a new level. Hahnemann and his successors restricted themselves over the course of two hundred years to the observation and description of phenomena. In the 1990's, an increasing number of homeopaths began, like Jan Scholten, to group and classify the Materia Medica not only in terms of elements and minerals, but also into remedies of plant and animal origin.

This step towards a cohesive system of its own is necessary for every scientific discipline, and it presents both advantages and disadvantages. On the one hand, it makes it possible to deduce a remedy's characteristics from its coordinate position, as shown in the example of *Germanium*. This also applies to physical symptoms, as far as they are group-specific. In this way many new remedies have come into use in recent years, much more quickly than through the classical method of proving substances on healthy persons. With these new remedies and with the method of group analysis, it is possible to help many patients who could not be cured using the conventional approach with better-known remedies. In many cases the homeopathic differential diagnosis becomes clearer and simpler. On the other hand, a degree of uncertainty and disorientation has initially been associated with this step to a new level of scientific awareness. In the transition phase from one step to the next, it is often difficult to distinguish between a working hypothesis that has not yet been confirmed, and established knowledge.

Therefore a homeopath should be well versed in the conventional method and well-known remedies before turning to new classification systems that are still in the process of development.

But now back to Wim. From a homeopathic viewpoint, his need for perfectionism and control is typically associated with remedies of metallic origin. However, Wim doesn't primarily want to control his environment. His motto is: "Whoever can conquer himself is stronger than someone who conquers an entire city." He is thus concerned with having control over himself. Throughout his life, he has lived according to his own laws. Being dependent on doctors or medications makes him depressed. This is why he says to the cardiologist: "It's my life and I decide." And he decides on a medical approach which supports his self-regulation. Jan Scholten connects this marked striving for independence and autonomy with the elements from the lanthanide series. The theme of this lateral arm of the sixth row of the periodic table, which was previously uncharted territory on the homeopathic map, also has to do with power and responsibility, but with an emphasis on self-control. Once Dr. Scholten had discovered this central theme for the homeopathic use of lanthanides in the course of his scientific research, he immediately thought of Wim.

In order to select one of these rare metals as a remedy for Wim, with the help of his coordinate system, Dr. Scholten still had to match Wim's typical reaction pattern to one of the eighteen vertical groups of this system. When we examine Wim's life story, we notice a certain urge to prove himself, to jump in at the deep end. Many minor anecdotes show that he already began looking for challenges in his childhood and never avoided conflicts. Scholten connects this behavior pattern with group six of his system. The lanthanide which falls into this group is the element with the atomic number 60, Neodymium (Nd). But we still have not quite reached our goal: The Dutch physician didn't prescribe the pure metal, but rather neodyme oxide. With the oxide component he takes into account another important theme in the life of his patient - the feeling of being treated unfairly, used and abused. The potentized *Neodymium oxydatum* is thus a remedy that is tailored to Wim - about as hard to find as the actual metal oxide in the earth's crust.

Even though neodyme has strong magnetic properties, it did not attract Dr. Scholten at the start. He initially selected various other remedies which addressed the problem areas Wim was confronted with at the time. The first remedy was also an oxide, since Wim was preoccupied at the beginning of his treatment with feeling exploited at work and cheated out of his patent. In Dr. Scholten's system, *Antimonium oxydatum* corresponds best to this type of problem. The dose of this homeopathic remedy not only decreased Wim's blood pressure, but also initiated a process which confronted Wim with his feelings, with old traumas and conflicts. His doctor accompanied him homeopathically on this journey into the past. With the exception of the goosefoot preparation used to treat his chronic otitis, Wim received only metallic remedies that each brought about a degree of success for certain complaints and problems. At the end of this clarification process, the neodyme oxide proved to be the constitutional remedy which brought the patient into a new equilibrium on all levels. His blood pressure was thus not reduced through a direct medicinal effect on his cardiovascular system (as with a beta blocker), but rather through the subtle homeopathic stimulation of the autoregulation of his whole organism. The result: Wim puts less pressure on himself.

9. Savita's Smile

> *As soon as you trust yourself, you will know how to live.*
>
> Johann Wolfgang von Goethe

Ravi was at the end of his rope. The three yards to the toilet right next to his bedroom on the second floor cost him his last ounce of strength. Bracing himself against the wall and on furniture, he pushed himself forwards inch by inch on his numb legs. He needed ten minutes to get there and ten minutes to get back from urinating, before he could fall back on his bed, exhausted. He absolutely refused to use a bedpan, although the doctors had recommended it to him. At least he could still make this decision for himself. A last scrap of human dignity left to him.

Downstairs in the kitchen, Savita heard the toilet flushing. She listened until the sound of feet dragging on the wood floor stopped and then gave him at least fifteen minutes, to be sure he had made it to his bed and recovered a bit. She took the bowl with the vegetable broth, which she had had to prepare for Ravi in the neighbor's kitchen. She was no longer allowed to cook in the house, because he couldn't stand the smell of food. It made him nauseous. And sometimes he vomited. Even though only bile and mucus could be forced out of his empty stomach. He would probably refuse the soup, just like everything else she had served him for many weeks. Nonetheless she didn't want to give up hope.

But she was afraid to go upstairs and see him in his misery. His sunken cheeks, the dark rings around his eyes. He would refuse to eat again. She forced herself to go upstairs to him anyway, then put on her smile and went into the bedroom. He was sleeping. And the smile vanished from her face.

His lower jaw hung down. He breathed heavily. Even when sleeping, he suffered from shortness of breath. She noticed the thick tongue twisted to the side. It hung out of his mouth, inflamed, covered with a thick white coating. A fungus had spread throughout his entire mouth. It had to be torture for him to sip water or tea. For weeks it had grown harder and harder for him to utter words. When he tried anyway, they came painfully and with incredible difficulty from his lips. One understood only fragments of what he babbled. Of course he knew that, and became more and more silent. The words also took away his air. Air that he needed to survive.

Everything was endlessly difficult for him: breathing, eating, excreting.

Savita crept out to the veranda which was attached to the bedroom. A giant banyan tree protected her there, with its thick roof of adventitious roots. From there she could observe Ravi's bed. Her husband had been suffering for six months from this terrible disease, whose name she had never heard before and could never remember. A rare autoimmune disease which could attack all the organs. So far only Ravi's nerves were affected. Only. His arms and legs felt dull and numb, he had such unbearable, splitting headaches, and he saw double. He would die soon, the doctors had told her, if he didn't take the poisonous medications. He would probably never be able to work again - that was their prognosis. And without the poison he had absolutely no chance. Savita would have to spend her last rupee on this costly treatment if she wanted to keep her husband alive. But what kind of a life was this? How long would he lie there like that?

Because his immune system turned against his own body and attacked it, it had to be suppressed with medications normally used in chemotherapy to fight tumors. The doctors in the hospital had explained this to her. The undesirable side effects – like these terrible headaches, the fungal infection and the insurmountable nausea – had to be accepted. There was no alternative. After he had been treated at the clinic twice as an inpatient, it was hoped that the medications would finally take effect. But his condition did not improve. Her already slender husband had lost almost fifty pounds. He looked pitiful. Savita dug the fingernails of her right hand into the palm of her left. She wasn't allowed to cry. She had to be strong. She had to give Ravi hope with her confidence and her smile. Again and again she reassured him, "Everything will be fine." She didn't tell him what she knew from the doctors about his illness and the prognosis. Everything was up to her. She had to find a way. She had to preserve the illusion of recovery for him, and at the same time pay for the expensive medical treatment and care for his mother, who lived with them, and for Raoul.

In two years their son would finish school. Going on to college, however, was now out of the question for Raoul, for he would be forced to work and support the family. Until then, Savita calculated, their savings could last. After that, there would probably be no choice but to sell Ravi's warehouse. She did not understand enough about the purchase and sale of gemstones to continue running the business alone, although he involved her in all of his business decisions and always asked for her advice. Ravi exported rough stones for jewelry-making to the USA, England and Central Europe. The diamond and gemstone trade held great risks and required a great deal of experience. Ravi had grown into his father's business, which the family had run for generations, but it still presented him again and again with financial worries. Although he had a sure touch for quality goods, fears plagued him constantly. He spent most of his time in the office, checking the quality of the stones, comparing the prices of his competitors, attending to long-standing customers and trying to win new ones. He could brood about business matters 24 hours a day, just as he now slept 24 hours a day.

While his father was alive, she understood his worries. It was not easy to work with the old man. And it was better to keep your mouth shut. Ravi tried incessantly to do everything the way he wanted. Sunil was the absolute ruler of the extended family. In business as well as in private life. He decided. With strictness and discipline. There was only one way to handle things. His. Ravi never argued with him. He was afraid of how his father would react. Ravi was most affected by the indifferent way his father could treat him. A certain amount of tension could not be completely avoided in the business or at home. Then he didn't speak to his son. He simply didn't acknowledge him. Ravi never knew what he was thinking, and he never asked him. Even though it hurt him that his father did not accept him, that he even rejected him, it was never brought out into the open. He couldn't discuss things with his father - Savita knew that. He put up with his father's moods as long as they lasted and then went on as before.

Her husband had had trouble making decisions during his entire life. But then his father had never encouraged him in any way. He didn't have any confidence in his quiet and gentle son. It had been that way since Ravi was a child. His father would like to have seen him roughhousing with other boys, playing wild games and doing sports, like boys were supposed to do. Instead Ravi drew a lot and read English literature. He was shy, reserved and taciturn. As a teenager, he had only one close friend he trusted. This friend had since moved to America and Ravi still missed him now. The second person he had been close to since childhood, his older sister, also no longer lived in Bombay. Savita was now his only support. With a happy smile, he sometimes told her how he had walked with his friend on stilts. As long and as far as possible. As soon as he stood up on the wooden slats he had carved himself, which extended his thin legs by yards like sturdy prostheses, he felt proud and exalted.

Ravi also conducted business in his quiet way. He never expressed his opinion; even if he was in favor of something, he never fought for it. Savita thought of the year when, on the advice of a business friend, Ravi wanted to deal more in emeralds, as the beautiful, green, velvety gemstones were becoming more and more rare and valuable. But his father didn't think much of the idea of specializing, and refused even to examine Ravi's selection of emeralds more closely. The two of them could not even reach a general agreement on the value of the largest and purest stone in the collection, although there were clear criteria for this. Ravi had given in as always, and he didn't even speak of the matter again when he found out that the business associate had become rich from the emerald trade. Such a reaction was typical for her husband. Not the least bit self-confident. She knew him intimately. And she loved him very much. That was why she stayed out of it. If she were Ravi, she would certainly have laid the numbers out on the table for Sunil.

One single time, Ravi summoned up his courage and argued with his father. Even though he had to pay for it for months by enduring his father's silent but obvious show of contempt, he didn't give in. Finally Sunil gave his son an ultimatum. He gave him a maximum of six months to leave the house and to run the company on his own account. He himself refused to continue working together with his son and no longer attended to the business matters he had previously managed single-handedly. He only took care of the old customers and turned them against his son. Ravi could soon feel their disapproval. He had to become acquainted with bookkeeping, administration and tax matters - areas he had no idea about, since he had been primarily responsible for sales and consulting. His father's brothers gave him tips from time to time. But this didn't really help him to manage the situation. The whole load was now on his shoulders. He could no longer concentrate on his work, although he thought of nothing else. The job made him sick. All of a sudden, he caught every infection and cold that was going around. On Savita's advice, he finally hired a qualified employee for the bookkeeping, which, as expected, caused more trouble with his father. For him it was clear once again that his son was a failure and never made any good decisions.

The ultimatum hung over Ravi like Damocles' sword. At times it seemed as though the entire matter had been forgotten, but still the threat loomed large in his mind. Where should he go? Why couldn't his father understand how impossible it was for him to leave his parents' house at 43 years of age? He was so attached to it. He was the only son. He belonged in this house. Sometimes his father appeared in his room in the middle of the night and icily demanded that he leave, preferably immediately.

A person denied support could end up having a complete breakdown. Ravi had met people who considered suicide when they missed a close relationship with their family. He would never go that far himself. He would do his best as long as it was somehow possible. He told himself that again and again. And he told Savita that too. As much as he tried, though, he couldn't oblige her by viewing the entire matter purely rationally. To have to leave his childhood home with his wife and son would have been a catastrophe for him. It wouldn't have meant just moving out, like any other adult finding an apartment and setting up home. Ravi absolutely could not imagine living and existing anywhere else. If his father threw him out of the house, there was no longer a safe place for him.

The cause of the dispute had to do directly with this house. Sunil swore by *Vastu Shastra*, the Indian form of *Feng Shui*, a 7000-year-old Vedic view of architecture in harmony with nature, the cosmos and energy fields. The four points of the compass play an important role in *Vastu*. Each direction supposedly carries and reinforces a certain potential for creativity, love and marriage, the health and finances of the house occupants. Sunil had various Swamis come into the house and make long lists of changes which were supposed to allow more energies, especially in the form of wealth, to flow into the rooms. The sticking point was Ravi's and Savita's bedroom in the southwestern section of the house. That was where his office should be in the future. But Savita absolutely did not want to give up this room. She loved the veranda and the mighty old banyan tree in front of it. It was her favorite place in the house. She loved to sit there with her husband. So Ravi said no. For the very first time. A reconciliation never did take place. He began halfheartedly to prepare for a possible move to the house of some distant relatives. Then his father died unexpectedly of a heart attack. Ravi could stay. But his health was affected. Maybe his severe illness had begun back then. In any case, his greatest fear after the death of his father was to become ill and bedridden, completely dependent on the help of others.

Savita! When Ravi awoke, he saw her through his half-opened eyes and thick lashes sitting on his bed. She was looking out of the window, where the evening sun sent its last ruby-colored rays into his bedroom. There was no smile on her face. The very smile that gave him hope of recovering. As long as Savita believed in him, nothing would happen. He remembered exactly how she had looked as a schoolgirl. He already loved her then, though it took him six whole years to propose to her. She was the only person he felt deeply attached to. She was his guardian angel. Besides her, there was no one else he could talk to. If Savita didn't smile anymore, it was over for him.

When she told him what she had decided, he consented immediately. Two young men from the neighborhood helped Savita carry her husband to the clinic of Dr. Jayesh Shah. They brought him into the small examining room and set him on a chair with sturdy armrests, so he wouldn't fall sideways. Ravi struggled to understand the doctor's questions. Between the few words he managed to utter, he had to gasp for air. When he didn't know an answer or was too exhausted, Savita spoke for him. This arduous procedure lasted for over two hours before Dr. Shah finally said, "I think I can help you." His assistant gave Savita a small envelope full of globules and exact instructions as to how she should dispense them. It was also her job to record every change in her husband's condition and report to Dr. Shah. Every day she phoned the doctor, and once a week she took Ravi to the clinic. On these occasions he announced, as always sparing with words, that he felt better. Yet it was his wife who observed in the many small aspects of daily life what enormous progress her husband was making. With her help, Dr. Shah was able to record an exact protocol of the healing process.

One week after beginning the homeopathic treatment, Ravi feels fresher, gets up in the mornings and even works briefly. After a temporary aggravation, the headaches have subsided. For the first time in months, he has a bit of an appetite. He eats rice with lentils and – Savita can hardly believe it – asks what there will be for dinner tomorrow. He would like pizza, and ice cream for dessert. He talks with visitors, watches television, walks around the house a few times. His mood is better. He takes his medicine himself, bathes alone and needs no help. Dr. Shah reduces by more than half the dosage of the medications which suppress Ravi's immune reaction.

A week later, Ravi takes part in family life again, goes out of the house and even drives the car himself. For the first time in a year. He now eats four small meals a day. He asks Savita to use plenty of condiments in her cooking, for he now likes his meals much spicier than before. He doesn't complain of pains anymore and Dr. Shah dares to stop one of the immune suppressants completely. The neurologist who examines Ravi regularly does not agree at all with this. He feels it is irresponsible to leave off the chemical medications and warns of the danger of brain or kidney damage. But Ravi relies completely on the intuition of his wife and on her doctor.

Another two weeks later, he feels fit and lively. Savita laughs when she tells Dr. Shah about him, because a few days before, Ravi had told her how he felt before the homeopathic treatment: "Like a wilted, withered vegetable." She tells him how happy she is to see her husband sitting on the veranda in the mornings, eating his breakfast and reading his business mail. He wants to start working more again and is feeling more adventurous. Yesterday they went on an outing for ten hours and he had no discomfort. His neurological test results have improved by 80 to 90 percent. The specialist still thinks it is a mistake to reduce or even stop his medications. He doesn't say a word about the homeopathy. One month later he feels vindicated, for Ravi suffers a relapse. He has severe headaches and sees double; the numbness in his legs has returned. Yet the specific laboratory test for this autoimmune disease shows no new disease activity.

The relapse remains a temporary setback in the healing process. Three months after beginning the homeopathic treatment, Ravi is stable again, and three months after that, he is almost completely healthy, except for a slight feeling of numbness in his right foot. He can work again, has more self-confidence, takes everything much more in his stride. The illness is behind him and he has the feeling that nothing more can happen to him. He reached his normal weight again some time ago. Nevertheless, he has bought himself some new clothes, fashionable and colorful. He doesn't feel like wearing black suits all the time anymore. And lately he has even been listening to loud music. Yes, he has really changed, says Savita; he has become more talkative and open and is not as diplomatic as he used to be. He knows what he wants and doesn't want, and he says so. He is now learning to enjoy life. Even though he still shares all of his thoughts and worries with her, he seems more independent and self-assured.

His new feeling in life is reflected in his dreams. After his death, his father had often appeared to him in his sleep, calming him and reassuring him that he would continue to support him in every way. Then he had laid his hand on the head of the son who bowed before him, and blessed him. Ravi had told Dr. Shah about this at the beginning of the treatment. Now he dreams again of his father. A large snake coils itself around his legs and has a stranglehold on him. Ravi jumps resolutely into action and sets his foot on the head of the snake. It uncoils itself immediately and slithers away. He is completely in control. This secure feeling of fearless determination accompanies him into the day upon awakening. He now knows that he can cope with even the most difficult situations. Now Dr. Shah finally tells him how terrible his illness really was, so dangerous that he could have died from it. And Savita smiles.

Commentary:

"We did not plan on you getting well again." With this sentence, Ravi's neurologist commented on his astonishing recovery from a disease that is considered incurable. Ravi suffered from mononeuritis multiplex, an inflammation of various nerves triggered in turn by an inflammation of the blood vessels supplying these nerves. The existence of the vascular disease behind the nerve disorder was indicated by special autoantibodies. These are antibodies of the immune system which can damage the body's own tissues. ANCA, an unusual antibody in Ravi's blood, is highly specific for a rare autoimmune disease of the blood vessels, known as Wegener's granulomatosis; this primarily affects the kidneys and lungs and is usually fatal if left untreated. And that was why the neurologist insisted on treatment with toxic medications, even though the potentially endangered organs were not – or not yet – affected by the disease.

In addition to high doses of cortisone, Ravi thus received cyclophosphamide, a cell toxin often used in cancer therapy, which suppresses the immune reaction of the organism. Due to its dreaded side effects, it is used in immune therapy only in life-threatening diseases. In Ravi's case it affected his stomach in particular. Because of the nausea, he was unable to eat anything for weeks, and when he finally came to Dr. Shah, he had already lost almost fifty pounds. At this time he was extremely weak and it was difficult to distinguish which part of his condition arose from the disease and which part from the ongoing treatment. Ravi was in any case certain that his condition had become considerably worse once he began taking the cyclophosphamide.

A state of therapeutic emergency is the term for such a situation, when conventional medicine has nothing more to offer and the patient often searches desperately for alternatives. As a rule, it is more often the patients than their doctors who ultimately turn to homeopathy. Many people do not come to a homeopathic practice until they have exhausted all of the possibilities of conventional treatment and their condition has not improved, but rather has worsened. The state of therapeutic emergency is a curse as well as a blessing for homeopathy. A curse, because all of the previous treatments can obscure the individual symptoms and interfere with the organism's ability to react, making it more difficult to find the right homeopathic approach. But also a blessing, because Hahnemann's successors are often called upon to treat severe illnesses and prove the potential of homeopathy even when the situation looks bleak, as with Ravi or when it is touch-and-go, as with Vijay in the case of "The Lost Warrior."

For a homeopathic understanding of Ravi and his remedy, it is helpful to compare his personality with that of the lost warrior. On the one hand, Mr. 100%, a strong and dominant self-made man who is totally sure of himself; on the other hand, the gentle, insecure and yielding Ravi, a total failure in the eyes of his father. The contrast between the two men could hardly be greater, and it is reflected in the homeopathic remedies which they received. For Vijay it was lead, one of the heaviest metals, at the very end of the row of stable elements in the periodic table. Ravi recovered with beryllium, one of the lightest metals, which is found near the very beginning of the periodic table as number four of the natural elements (see the Glossary). It is extracted from the gemstone beryl, which occurs in various colors. Ravi is well acquainted with its green and blue variations, the emerald and the aquamarine.

Dr. Jayesh Shah has occupied himself extensively with the application of the periodic table in homeopathy. In his opinion, there is a correlation between a person's self-esteem, that is to say the "weight" of his ego, and the atomic weight of the chemical element needed as a homeopathic remedy. Vijay's extremely strong ego corresponds to the heavy lead in the sixth row of the periodic table; a light metal from the second row fits Ravi's low self-confidence. According to Dr. Shah and the Bombay school of homeopathy, the remedies in this second row are concerned with the development of one's own, still weakly pronounced individuality. *Beryllium* is located right near the beginning of this row, in the second vertical group of the periodic table. To this group of so-called alkaline earth metals belong the often-prescribed elements magnesium, calcium and barium. The emotional symptoms shared by these remedies revolve around such themes as insecurity, giving way to others, passivity, a need for protection, dependence on the support of others, lack of confidence, and sensitivity to being observed. In *Beryllium*, the entire complex of ego weakness is most distinct and Dr. Shah clearly recognized the typical pattern of this remedy in Ravi.

There is definitely a similarity between Ravi's physical condition and some symptoms of the remedy proving of *Beryllium*, such as nausea, lack of appetite, emaciation, extreme weakness and shortness of breath on the least effort. In his prescription, however, the physician relied primarily on the strong correspondence in terms of the characteristic personality traits. Our case histories show how important it is, especially in severe illnesses, to comprehend the core of a person's problems, the central disturbance which runs like a thread through the person's life.

In Ravi's case, it was the feeling of inferiority and dependence. Because he was worthless in the eyes of his father, he did not believe he could not stand on his own two feet. It is significant for him that he loved to walk on stilts as a child. Throughout his entire life, he needed support. And he was always afraid of losing this and being turned out of the security of his parents' house. He couldn't imagine leading a family and a business on his own, without the support of his father. After the death of his father, he lived in constant fear of becoming unable to work and bedridden, until exactly that came to pass. His central disturbance, his inner state, manifested itself externally in a severe illness which left him totally dependent and helpless. He fought against this and dragged himself to the toilet unaided, to preserve his last bit of dignity. And in his wife he had a support who – in contrast to his father - cared for him with love. Yet the position he had assumed and become accustomed to in life remained the same. Until his encounter with *Beryllium*.

In engineering, this element is used against "metal fatigue". Although it is not particularly hard, it lends hardness to other elements and alloys, so that they can withstand loads better. Analogous to this, potentized *Beryllium* proved to be an inner support for Ravi. Dr. Shah gave it to him after the first consultation in the C 200 potency, and repeated the remedy every time he reduced the cortisone dosage. Here he was very prudent, and only cut back the immunosuppressive therapy as far as the condition of his patient allowed. In the case of such a severe autoimmune disease, it is necessary to follow a dual-track policy and not just abruptly discontinue the current medications. The reduction of the immunosuppressives depends on the course of the symptoms, laboratory tests and other clinical results which are typical for the disease.

In order to estimate the specific effect of the homeopathic remedy, it is necessary, however, to consider the reactions of the organism on all levels, particularly in the field of the central disturbance. Only when something changes here, only when *Beryllium* can balance out the deficit which is typical for this person and his remedy, is it possible to reckon on a lasting recovery. Therefore Dr. Shah was not fully satisfied with the course of the treatment until he observed how Ravi became more self-confident and independent, allowing him to achieve a new sense of freedom in his life. After this clear change in his inner attitude and his outlook on life, it is no surprise that Ravi has been healthy now for seven years and has not suffered any relapse of this dreadful disease.

10. A Part of the Family

> *Smiling is the most elegant way to bare your teeth to the enemy.*
>
> *Werner Finck*

Sonja, a magnificent and regal figure and the heroine of this story, is very punctual for the appointment early in the morning in Bombay. It is important for her to explain first her very special relationship to her homeopathic physician: "Dr. Sujit calls me Didi. Sister. My doctor is like a brother for me and the favorite uncle of my children, so I call him Mama – my mother's brother. He has thousands of patients and is part of the family everywhere. But the relationship between the two of us comes from the heart. You can't buy love – with money you can buy everything, but not love. I have always helped him, even when he had big problems himself. He knew he could call Didi anytime and she would come, even in the middle of the night."

Her doctor, Sujit Chatterjee, smiles as he adjusts her chair and reminds his "adopted sister" of their first meeting 15 years ago. "That is true, Didi. Since you came to my practice, you have been part of the family. You entertained my visitors back then. Do you remember? But wasn't there also a small dispute?"

Sonja probably wouldn't have mentioned it, but she hasn't forgotten. "Sujit Mama, back then you were a bit more interested in your visitors than in me." Today they can both laugh about it.

That the doctor and his patient would one day address each other with the terms of endearment "favorite uncle" and "honored older sister" could not really have been foreseen then, for the first encounter between "Sujit Mama" and "Sonja Didi" in Dr. Chatterjee's medical practice was anything but friendly. Sonja and her sick child arrived a quarter hour before the scheduled appointment, and the eight-year-old was screaming blue murder. After she observed for ten minutes with growing indignation from the waiting room how the doctor sat in the next room talking to some visitors, pouring them tea and offering sweets, she lost patience. She pushed the door open, took hold of the teapot and demanded that the doctor please attend immediately to her sick child. In the meantime she would take care of his visitors. They could certainly wait a while, but not her son, who was in agony.

Dr. Sujit Chatterjee didn't hesitate a second, and immediately examined the child, who was obviously suffering from meningitis. During the examination, Sonja took wonderful care of the visitors with a friendly smile. However, the strangers who had stolen Sonja's time with the doctor weren't just anyone, but his future parents-in-law. Though Sonja wasn't to know that back then. Fortunately the relatives of the bride weren't ones to bear a grudge. The doctor wasn't either and so, he says with a delicate smile, "This is how Sonja became a part of the family from the beginning." He has not escaped from Sonja's care since then. She loves to cook his favorite meals for him, makes sures everything is running smoothly in the practice when he is away and maintains her friendly relationship to her doctor and his household with sincere affection and love. To ensure he is completely cared for, she prays twice a day in the temple for the gods to bless him.

Sonja knows exactly why she swears by Sujit Mama. He helped her son and also her husband, the police officer. After a recurrent herniated disk, which caused him so much discomfort that he limped, he was finally free of pain thanks to Dr. Sujit's homeopathic treatment and could show off his impressive figure to advantage, as was proper for a public officer. A police officer who cannot stand up straight while walking the streets – unimaginable!

No, it wasn't funny back then. Even though her husband Ray has a very good sense of humor. For many years he has cultivated his inner cheerfulness as an active member of a laughing yoga club. There he practises together with other people "sincere laughter," "lion laughter" or "one-yard laughter." It is very good for her husband. She doesn't need it herself; she finds her well-being in religion. Back then, when she had the accident, she was only accompanying him to the laughter club picnic for members and their spouses. The evening ended badly and marked the beginning of a crisis for Sonja.

It happened on the way home: Sonja fell on the rainy street and landed hard on the back of her head. For a few seconds, she could see only darkness around her and couldn't even remember her own name. Afterwards her head hurt terribly for days, as if someone were pulling her brains out. Over the next two weeks, the pain became so severe that she vomited several times. She felt worst when sitting. Even when she poured a bucket of water over her head, it didn't get better. It helped a little to bend her head forward, but most of the time she had to lie down.

On the day of the Divali Festival in October 1998, when she was actually supposed to visit her husband's relatives, Sonja called her doctor and favorite uncle and told him about the unbearable headaches which came in waves and made daily life impossible, so that she could not cope with her work at home or at the office. Even simple things such as going to the toilet in the morning or brushing her teeth were unthinkable. It appeared to be a severe concussion. But the headache did not come from Sonja's fall. The CT revealed a completely different and shocking diagnosis: a small meningioma, a benign tumor of the meninges, sat at the septum pellucidum between the two halves of the brain. Because of the terrible headaches, the doctors in the hospital advised an immediate operation, for them the only possible therapy in this situation. But Sonja wanted to be treated homeopathically by her uncle. She trusted him completely. He could cure her son's meningitis and her husband's herniated disk, so there was no reason why he couldn't bring the meningeal growth under control.

Dr. Chatterjee was distraught about the misfortune that had befallen his honored older sister. He had recently lost his first wife to cancer and he had become very fond of Sonja as a friend, over the eight years he had known her. For Sonja the word "tumor" naturally also triggered terrible fears. Who should look after her children, who were only 16 and 17, if she died? Of course they noticed that their mother could not even walk in a straight line, never mind cook or work at her job. They saw how apathetic Sonja was and they feared for her life. Sonja herself told her doctor that she was only thinking of the others when she thought of her death. If it really came to get her, she would say, "Death! Wait another 10 years! Not yet!"

Well, it would not come to that. Sujit explained to Sonja the difference between a malignant brain tumor and her benign meningioma. It wasn't directly life-threatening, but it could grow and ultimately impair important brain functions. As yet, however, no immediate danger existed and there was time to wait for the effects of his homeopathic treatment. The operation was postponed and Dr. Chatterjee initially prescribed potentized *Platinum*, a remedy which had proved helpful for Sonja in the past. But the precious metal had no impact on her unbearable headaches and her desperate condition. The doctor therefore had to retake Sonja's case, ask her again about her sensations and perceptions in life and pay special attention to finding out anything new about her.

He already knew a lot about her. When she was just 15 years old, she was forced as a girl to leave home in Gujarat in the northwest of India because there wasn't enough income to support the entire family. Her father, the only person in Sonja's eight-member household who earned any money, was an alcoholic. And Sonja was terribly ashamed of the way her father behaved when he was drunk, how he screamed or made a fool of himself in front of others. A father was supposed to be a decent man who knew how to behave and was respected by everyone. She never forgave him for his bad behavior. Or for throwing her out of the house. Because one of her older sisters was very gifted, the father had decided that she could continue to attend school and Sonja should go off and earn money. She was sent to an uncle in Bombay.

She felt like a stranger in the new extended family in which she lived, but never belonged. She was not treated the same as her cousins: she had to get up very early, help her aunt with the lavish Indian cuisine, wash the clothes and clean the house. Afterwards she worked all day at a pharmacy, cut herbs and spices, filled jars with rose petals and honey, washed out the bottles and measured and sealed the medicine packages. Her daily wage was 75 rupees – about two dollars today. And even though she knew that she couldn't expect a better job with her mediocre education, she felt that the work she had to do was beneath her dignity and dreamed of a career as a stewardess in a pretty uniform. Smiling sweetly and charmingly was part of behaving perfectly and she also practised this in her uncle's house. Not because she felt it in her heart, but because she was always afraid of being thrown out. She obeyed as well as she could. She didn't feel better until later, when she found work in a telephone company, earned good money and in time became their receptionist. Today, after more than thirty years, she feels like the mother of the company, even though she started at the bottom back then, just after she married.

Sonja served for seven years in her uncle's house, before she married Ray at the age of 22. It was an arranged marriage. She was led to the house of the potential groom and his parents, judged by her prospective husband and told after a week that the young man had fallen for her. In accordance with convention, Sonja was from the same caste, had the same religious practices and holidays, the same cooking and eating habits. At first she was proud of her husband, the police officer; she loved uniforms so much and, moreover, he was good-looking and nice. Ray's excessive sexual drive didn't become a problem until later on. Sonja knew little about physical love and had to learn about it through smutty magazines that were only available under the counter in shady kiosks. They had titles such as "69 Tips for a Wife to Make Her Husband Happy in Bed." Sonja was determined to be a perfect wife. And so she devotedly gave him everything a loving wife owed her spouse. Even twice a day, if that was what he desired.

But inside she felt terrible and she became more and more convinced that this family was beneath her. From the beginning there was trouble between Sonja and her parents-in-law; this went far beyond the disputes between mother-in-law and daughter-in-law that are normal in India. Ray's mother was strict, narrow-minded and domineering. Sonja, on the other hand, tried to be devoted, patient and demure. She endured everything out of love for her husband. If she raised her voiced only slightly, the old woman cut her short. When she became pregnant in the first year as expected, and asked for time to rest, they made her keep working. Because her husband earned too little, she had to continue working in the office. When she came home exhausted in the evening, all of the housework was waiting for her. Sonja got up at five in the morning to cook ahead for the day. For the meal had to be on the table on time in the evening, otherwise there was no end to her mother-in-law's tirades. Her father-in-law, and unfortunately also her husband, usually joined in too.

When Sonja was sick during the second pregnancy, her mother-in-law didn't even provide her with food. The relationship didn't get any better as the children grew older. Because she wanted them to be brilliant in school, Sonja coached them a lot. Ray and his parents found this unnecessary, however. Sonja's priorities were supposed to be taking care of the household and her in-laws, and when she continued to put her children first, there were arguments, ructions and accusations. She didn't defend herself; she said nothing about it all and cried only in secret. Soon there were more bitter pills to swallow in this exemplary marriage. It was the last thing she would have expected. Her husband, of all people, started to drink. She had always wanted a respectable husband, with very good English and perfect manners. Everyone should ask, "Whose husband is *that*?" His impeccable behavior and his flawless appearance should have ennobled Sonja as his wife. Even when Ray maintained he only had the occasional glass with colleagues or friends at parties, it made her extremely angry. She insisted on total abstinence. If he really loved her, he wouldn't touch a drop of alcohol. He was drinking and wasting away her love. And if a man had any regard for the character and dignity of his wife, he would not constantly demand sex from her. Ray didn't want to go a single day without sex. He didn't want anything else from her. Even after 17 years of marriage. It remained a contentious issue in their relationship and Sonja was certainly not a woman to suffer in silence. She reproached him about it all again and again: the drinking, his sexual addiction, his bad manners, his nasty parents. But never in front of others. Not in front of the relatives or neighbors. Not in front of the in-laws. Not in front of the children. Everyone should think that Ray was the love of her life and that she was a saint, the ideal wife and daughter-in-law.

She would much rather her husband didn't go out on his own or with buddies. She just didn't like that. He should only be seen in public with her. To prove how important she was to him. But discreetly. Ray just didn't understand that. Sonja gave her doctor an example: Recently Ray was driving home with her in the evening. It was already dark, and he kissed her in the car. Sonja was horrified. You just didn't do things like that. It wasn't normal to show affection in public. Even young couples holding hands were frowned upon. How could Ray kiss her in front of everyone? Sujit had to laugh. He found it totally normal for a man to kiss his own wife in the dark. There was nothing wrong with that. Why was she so extremely sensitive about improper behavior, as she saw it? But Sonja didn't think there was anything funny about it. She was deeply hurt. People could think she was cheap. She was proud of being able to see all of this and talk about it so clearly and uncompromisingly. She was the perfect wife. And in comparison to her, Ray was a nobody. That was exactly what she had slung at him. And then he got mean.

That time, Ray didn't stick to appeasing her and calming her down like he usually did, by saying, "Cool down Baby, cool down!" He became angry, yelled at her and accused her of being domineering and telling him what to do, just like she did with the children. She just didn't give people any freedom and if she kept on like this, he would throw her out sometime. "Beat it!" he would say. "Get out of here!" That hit her hard.

When Sonja told Sujit the story about the kissing in the car and her husband's outrageous reaction, she was full of indignation and absolutely unwilling to see the situation from another perspective. Sujit noticed more clearly than before how unreasonable and selfish she could be, and how condescendingly she could talk about her husband, while at the same time swearing she loved him above all else. It became clear to him how important appearances were to her. Ray shouldn't make a spectacle of himself and no one should point their finger at her. She was extremely disappointed in her husband. He didn't love her the way she wanted him to. So why did she stay with him anyway? Why didn't she say no when he demanded too much sex from her? Sonja Didi sobbed when Sujit Mama asked her so directly. She carried a great torment inside of her. If she didn't let him do what he wanted, she explained, he would go to one of those "ladies". To a prostitute. That would be the most terrible thing that could happen to her. Then all she had invested in her love would be for nothing. She would lose the respect of society. Her reputation and that of her children would be completely destroyed if word got around. And that would inevitably happen if her husband sneaked off to such a woman.

Sujit understood Sonja a bit more after this confession. He saw how she wanted to change her husband, who she didn't feel was worthy of her, through her love. He grasped how much effort she made and how hard she worked for her family, recognizing in this behavior her yearning for attention and her fear of being cast out. At this point she was stuck. In 17 years of marriage, nothing had changed and her husband still didn't appreciate her. Not a single gift in all this time. No positive word about her. He never defended her, not even when his mother came at her with outrageous accusations, for example that she met other men instead of going to the office. And misappropriated money that belonged to the whole family. Sonja had denied this, deeply hurt. Everyone could see how carefully she cleaned and cared for her only two saris. She was content with just one lipstick. She never went to a beauty salon like other young women. She never bought anything for herself. She earned thousands of rupees, but the money she was allowed to keep for herself was just enough to pay for the monthly ticket for the public transportation she took to the office. Mother got the rest.

But Mother was never satisfied. What more did she want, anyway? Sonja didn't complain about the ridiculous amount of 50 rupees she was allowed per month as pocket money. She swallowed the constant criticism. She stuck it out, took wonderful care of the household and the in-laws, raised the children according to strict principles, and greeted her husband every day – in spite of everything – with a smile on her lips and a glass of water for him.

Why did she do all of this?

"Ray didn't want to see any long faces when he came home, and I did it all just for him, because I was so happy with my husband and wanted to make him happy too. It was supposed to be like seventh heaven!"

Sonja affirmed this again and again, although she was surely aware her doctor knew the other side of the story. But he kept quiet and let her speak.

"Keep yourself happy!" That had always been her motto, she said. "You can't change the other person, only yourself." So she acted in accordance with her motto. "Be nice to your husband and also to your parents-in-law, respect them! That will please them. Maybe not today. Maybe not tomorrow. But one day they will notice."

But the truth was, they didn't notice. Never in all of these years. They didn't give Sonja the attention she wished for. They didn't praise her. Mother would always be a shrew. Ray didn't give her the love she craved. And her father-in-law was an indecent person. He had no idea of what was proper, just like Ray. He stood around all the time in the tiny kitchen when she was cooking for the family, taking up space and reading his newspaper. She hated the very smell of his newspaper. She always had to squeeze past him and push him aside, so he wouldn't touch her and so she wouldn't get caught on him with her round hips. There were men who liked to paw women. Sonja immediately sensed with men when there was something untoward in the atmosphere. Then she would speak up loud and clear, even with her father-in-law.

It was simply unthinkable that another man could be allowed to touch her. If any man tried it, she would break all of his bones. She carried a stick to defend herself against indecent overtures in the crowded streets of the city. She had absolutely no interest in other men. That was why she was so outraged at the insinuation that she played around. For that, she would love to have slapped her mother-in-law across the face.

Dr. Sujit believed her outrage, but he also knew another truth. Sonja had confessed it to him herself, when he was looking for a new remedy for her and her tumor. There had, in fact, been an encounter with another man. He worked in the same company. Sonja and this man had become friends and talked a lot with each other about his unhappy marriage. His wife had to be the opposite of Sonja. That meant the most imperfect wife one could possibly imagine. She couldn't even cook. For her new friend, Sonja solicitously brought home-cooked food to the office. They became closer. Of course she didn't tell Ray anything about this budding relationship. She "taught this friend" (as she put it to her doctor and favorite uncle) "how to love a wife. It was a gift. For his wife too." However, someone from the company called this wife and told her about Sonja's lavish care for her husband. He withdrew. Very well-behaved and discreet. So there would be no scandal, either in his marriage or in Sonja's. But Sonja was not thankful toward this gentleman. She was extremely angry and hurt. How could he dare to reject her, to disregard her love? Was she just dirt or rubbish?

It was her old trauma: being cast out and ignored. Sujit understood her strong wish to belong, to be important, to play a significant role in the lives of others. He could see how happy it made her to be seen as his "sister" and to be a part of his family. Belonging and being in the middle of it all made her proud and content. The thought of being excluded made her panic. Even greater than the anger toward her in-laws and her husband was the fear that she could be thrown out of her house. This fear had accompanied her throughout her life, since she was forced to leave her parents' house at 15.

Dr. Chatterjee was already familiar with all of these aspects of the patient he knew so well, but they now formed a new picture. He no longer saw in her the precious and hard platinum, but rather a beautiful and delicate plant, the meadow saffron. Just a few weeks after taking the first dose, Sonja Didi had everything under control again – her family, her job, her household. The headaches were gone and never returned. And along with them, the meningioma disappeared. A little less than two years later, the radiologist could find no trace of the tumor in the magnetic resonance image. He also searched in vain for a surgical scar and was surprised, when he looked at the old images of Sonja's brain, how exceedingly healthy and trim this woman appeared in her expensive new silk sari.

Not only the sari was new. In Sonja's life, a lot of things had changed in these two years. She observed the behavior of her husband with unusual tolerance. She let him go to parties and forgave him when he drank now and then. After all, it wasn't a catastrophe. She was responsible for her own behavior and he for his; she realized that now. And so she simply accepted him as he was. She gave him and others more leeway and didn't make a big deal about a faux pas anymore. When Ray was transferred by the government to Kashmir, she took it calmly. Previously she would not have been able to imagine a life without her husband. Today she wouldn't say that anymore. She enjoys her independence and her life with her two adult children and can look after herself very well. Her husband knows that now. He only comes home every two to six months for vacations.

Sonja finally has her own realm now. A place where she makes all the decisions. For she has bought a new house, financed mainly with money she earned herself. For tax reasons, it is listed in her name, with the consent of her husband. The in-laws do not live in Sonja's new house. How is this possible?

They said when they packed their belongings, "Sonja, you have cared for us loyally and devotedly in every way for 19 years. We feel it's time for you to have a somewhat easier life, so now we are moving to live with our second son and his wife."

At these words Dr. Sujit, who returns after leaving the room for a while, simply smiles delicately and quietly. Maybe they did say it a bit differently, says Sonja. Not quite the way she would have wished. They didn't want to live with her and Ray anymore. It probably offended their sense of honor to live in a house that didn't belong to their son, but to their daughter-in-law. Incidentally, Sonja comments, Ray's parents are being treated very badly by their second son and his wife. She has heard that directly from her mother-in-law. She explained recently how Sonja had been the backbone of the house, the family and their entire lives. Sonja's worth is finally recognized. Fine. But too late.

Is it perhaps possible that she actually threw her in-laws out of the house, wonders Dr. Sujit, the same way they had wanted to do to Sonja? He thinks he can remember her pointedly placing their suitcases in front of the door. No, she counters, she would never do something like that, for it is to them she owes her husband, who she loves so much and wants to make happy. Her own feelings are insignificant in comparison. But all of these thoughts are unnecessary, thank the Lord Krishna, because the in-laws – however it happened – are gone and she has told the visitors from Germany her whole story, which she had previously confided only in her beloved doctor, for only one reason: because of her heartfelt thankfulness toward Sujit Mama, whose homeopathy made her meningioma disappear and helped her become a happy and satisfied woman.

After Sonja has left, Sujit ventures a prognosis. If it turned out that the in-laws were even more unhappy at the brother's and Ray suggested that they move back in, she would simply say, "Sorry, baby. Out of the question." And Ray would keep quiet, call a few buddies and go with them to the laughter club and then allow himself a few beers afterwards. Sonja, in a perfectly fitting sari and with her most tender and loving smile on her lips, would wave good-bye to him, in clear view of the neighbors, until he was no longer within earshot of her jingling bracelets.

Commentary:

Another miraculous story of healing from India. First a herniated disk with symptoms of paralysis, then a life-threatening autoimmune disease and now even a meningioma, a tumor that puts pressure on the brain. Can such serious illnesses simply disappear without operations, radiation or strong medications? They certainly can, say even critics of homeopathy. After all, there are recorded cases of spontaneous healing among cancer patients. This is the usual term, reserved in conventional medicine for astonishing recoveries that cannot be scientifically explained; the term can certainly be applied, from a scientist's point of view, to every single case in this book.

Spontaneous means "coming from the inside, from a sudden inner drive, involuntarily, with no external stimulus". This type of healing actually takes place every second of our lives, a daily miracle which eludes our perception. For we usually do not notice how our organism constantly works to maintain its balance and regenerate itself. We quickly become impatient, however, when it doesn't happen to work so well. Yet every small injury and every slight infection gives us the opportunity to experience spontaneous healing for ourselves. In comparison to this healing which comes from inside, every medication and medical intervention is second-rate. We do not need a physician unless the self-healing forces of our inner physician are not working as they should or as we would like them to - when spontaneous healing does not take place fast enough or does not take place at all.

While conventional medicine pursues the strategy of replacing the inner physician with an outside agent to repair and control the organism, homeopathy (in common with other regulative methods of natural medicine) continues to trust in the potential of self-healing. Since this does not always take place spontaneously, it must sometimes be helped along with a precise stimulus, a specific piece of information. The success of a homeopathic treatment is thus distinguishable from the phenomenon of spontaneous healing in only one point: Healing does not take place without an external stimulus.

Of course in individual cases we never know exactly what would have happened without the impulse of the globules. Perhaps Sonja's meningioma would have disappeared anyway, through spontaneous healing. But Dr. Chatterjee didn't trust to luck. He had clear criteria for the prescription of a homeopathic remedy and for judging the progress of his treatment. And he had enough time to wait for the remedy to act, since the slow-growing tumor was benign. He would never have taken a risk. After all, Sonja was like a sister to him. But for this very reason, it was not so easy to find the optimal remedy for her. He had known her for a long time, had a clear picture of her and had successfully prescribed Platinum in the past on the basis of this picture.

We have repeatedly encountered people in this book who were cured homeopathically with heavy metals. Like Sonja, they were performance-oriented, ambitious, perfectionist and had a strong ego. Sonja's regal appearance is typical of "Platinum women", who tend to think they are something special and are known among homeopaths for their arrogance and dominance. Rajan Sankaran writes about this remedy type: "Platinum is the 'queen' –she must carry herself regally, show herself superior....The expectation felt by [her] is to be something special – a level of performance much above normal." And of course she also expects her husband and children to fulfil these same high standards. Her attitude toward sexuality is ambivalent: On the one hand, her majesty would like to stand above such base instincts. But on the other hand, her feeling of superiority is bound up with her attractiveness to the male sex.

Significant aspects of Sonja's character matched this personality profile of the Platinum woman and the metal had thus far proved useful as a remedy for her. It had no influence, however, on the unbearable headaches.

Dr. Chatterjee therefore looked for a new remedy that was similar to *Platinum*, but also addressed the aspects of his patient and her illness not covered by the precious metal. Here the doctor made use of a method of questioning developed by Dr. Sankaran, and tried through understanding her main symptom to find a common denominator for Sonja's physical complaints and her conspicuous psychological characteristics. Throughout her biography, there was a central theme of feeling cast out, first from her parents' house, then from her relatives' home and finally from her own household. She always lived in fear of being pushed out. In the way she described her headaches, Dr. Chatterjee now discovered a very similar picture: as though someone were pulling her brains out with force. Here was the key to the homeopathic remedy, as this feeling of being "cast out, pushed out or pulled out" directly expressed the central disturbance of the vital force on the physical, emotional and mental levels. Rajan Sankaran speaks in such a case of the "vital sensation." In recent years, he has classified botanical families according to their vital sensations and established a coordinate system for homeopathic plant remedies similar to that developed by Jan Scholten for the chemical elements. Sonja's particular pain, as an expression of her vital sensation, led her doctor first to the lily family, and with the help of Sankaran's system, he then selected the remedy Colchicum from this group of plants.

This assignment to the lilies is not solely attributable to the vital sensation. In the experience of many homeopaths, people whose similes are lilies place a great deal of importance on their outer appearance, on respect, on their social position and on perfect behavior. With their high standards, they can seem arrogant and can be easily confused with the *Platinum* type. Behind a facade of morality and perfectionism, they hide their fear of being cast out. Like Sonja, they try very hard to belong and are willing to endure a great deal in their family, partnership and profession. Their care and efforts for others are in direct contrast to the remedy picture of Platinum.

For the remedy *Colchicum*, Sonja's personal lily, the sensitivity toward bad behavior, toward faux pas in public, is especially typical (and the plant's folk name of 'naked ladies' in several European languages has interesting parallels here.) However there were also physical symptoms which indicated the need for the meadow saffron. Above all, the pronounced sensitivity to smell during the headaches was an indication for *Colchicum*, as was the unusual relief of the pain on bending over. But because this plant was chosen not just for Sonja's headaches, but as a much deeper-acting remedy for her primal fear of being cast out, it had to demonstrate its effectiveness in this area as well. The essential effect of the homeopathic treatment therefore showed itself for Dr. Chatterjee in the psychological change in his Sonja Didi. She became more relaxed and tolerant toward her family and at the same time better able to fulfill her own needs.

This new inner freedom is the true sign of the homeopathic cure. The fact that in Sonja's case a meningioma vanished into thin air at the same time – whether spontaneously or not - is an exceedingly gratifying side effect.

11. The Poison of Fear

> *"Heinrich, the carriage is breaking apart!"*
> *"No master, the carriage it is not;*
> *It is a band that encased my heart*
> *As it suffered so*
> *When you sat in a well*
> *And were changed into a frog"*
>
> The Brothers Grimm (The Frog Prince)

Adam is afraid. If he doesn't fight it, his eyes will close, he will go to sleep and his mother will leave him too, without him noticing. That's why he must keep on calling her - and she must answer. Then he hears her voice and knows she is still there. For now! But any minute she could be gone. So he must call to her again. Every few minutes. He hears her clattering the crockery in the kitchen and she says loudly, "Yes Adam, I'm here." But is it really Klara his mother who is talking to him? He wants to be sure - she must come to his bedside. Adam is in despair. His heart hurts. He has bound a belt around his chest - so tight that it is cutting into him. He needs the band around his body because he is afraid that his heart will burst with the pain.

Six years ago when the pregnancy test showed positive and Adam announced his presence, his mother was not at all certain that this was the right time to have a child. Klara's new relationship was only a few months old and her partner Ben, a few years younger than herself, was at the start of a new university course. Her stressful, underpaid job as a freelance landscape gardener was neither safe nor paying her social security. What would they live on? Klara decided to keep her baby in spite of this and when he was born, all the problems solved themselves. After a short while, Klara was offered a permanent part-time job and Ben got a grant which gave his studies a fairly solid financial footing. In addition to this, Ben, light-footed lover of life that he was, proved himself to be a loving and sweet father. He organized his studies so that he could look after his little son while Klara went to work. And in the big old house that they shared with other young people there was always someone who could baby-sit for the evening now and then. There was also room for a second child. A year after Adam, his little sister Lilly was born.

Klara was happy for three years. Then came a huge shock. Without warning, Ben suddenly left her for another woman.

The children were also stunned and bewildered. Daddy, who they loved so much, didn't love Mummy any more, but loved a lady from the next village and that was why he was suddenly gone. Every week they drew red dots on the calendar and waited impatiently until the days with the blue dots - days with Daddy - finally came around. Saying goodbye to him was incredibly difficult for them every time. After two years, however, Adam and Lilly had learned that even though Daddy didn't want to live with Mummy, he was nearby and they could see him regularly. In the meantime, Klara had found Jonas, a cheerful man who was completely reliable. The children also experienced the light-hearted peace and security which he gave her. They liked Jonas from the word go. But just as everything was running smoothly, Ben topped it all by announcing that he had accepted a job in a large scientific project in Argentina. In effect, this meant that apart from a few exceptions, Ben would not come to Germany for three years.

Nothing to worry about, said Ben. Klara could put the kids on a plane when they wanted to visit him. A 32-hour flight with three changes at 800 Euros a head. They'd find someone to accompany them somehow. For Ben it was all no problem but Adam's world collapsed. It was shortly before his sixth birthday and in his intelligent little head he had already realized that it just wouldn't work out. As always, he had to know every detail. How many miles would there be between him and his Daddy? How long would the flight there take? How often would Klara be able to afford tickets? When were you allowed to be absent from school and for how long? How much holiday would Ben have from the project? And so on and so forth. The answers made it clear to him that his father would not just pop by for his birthday or to celebrate his first day at school. Daddy had always said that the separation from Mummy had nothing to do with him and that he loved his only son more than anything else. He would never desert him but would always and for ever be there for him. Even if it rained cats and dogs. But that was all lies. Ben had left him!

Adam was in despair. Whilst his sister Lilly cried and howled for hours every night until she was blue in the face (but then allowed herself to be comforted and went to sleep) he pulled himself together. After all, he was nearly old enough to go to school and he wanted to be brave. Nobody should see how much he missed Daddy. So he withdrew. When the other boys played outside, he wasn't interested. He didn't go outside any more. He didn't even want to visit his friend Paul, who lived nearby. He also didn't want Paul's mother to fetch him by car. He didn't trust her and wouldn't get in the car with her any more - or in Annie's car either, a neighbor who often gave him a lift to kindergarten. Both women liked Adam a lot and he had known them for a long time, but still he couldn't be persuaded to go with them. He'd rather not play. Nothing could tempt him, not even birthday parties or trips to the swimming pool.

Adam would not leave Klara's side. He would not go into another room if his mother didn't go with him. He didn't want to see anyone any more. When he lay in bed in the evening, all the doors had to be open. Klara and Jonas were not allowed out of earshot. Adam called out to Klara over and over again - more and more frequently and ever more pitifully, from eight in the evening until midnight. Each time she had to answer him at length, soothingly and gently so he could hear and absorb her voice. He cried and whimpered up to thirty times an hour, even when Klara and Jonas had friends round and the murmur of voices was easily heard in the boy's room. It wasn't enough for Adam to simply hear his mother talking like that - she had to answer him. She had to come, sit on his bed and hold his hand.

He wouldn't allow himself to go to sleep and kept himself awake for up to three hours at a time while Klara and Jonas stood by his bed. They assured him with all the promises they could think of that they wouldn't go away and that there was no reason for him to be afraid. They continually showed him that they were near, went into his room when he called, sat by his side, got up in the night and comforted him constantly and patiently. But still he was consumed by fear. In the end it wasn't even enough to sleep in their bed. Adam tied a rope to Klara's foot and clung to the other end. He kept his big blue eyes open and propped up the lids with his fingers if they fell shut with fatigue.

I must not sleep. I must not - no way. He sat up in bed and screamed, "I'm scared, I'm scared, I'm scared!" Klara tried tenderness, tried stories and tried to reason with him. But Adam's answer to any comforting or explanations was: "If I close my eyes, you'll go away."

Nothing got through to him - he had an answer to every argument. Even the fact that all the doors were open in the evening and he could hear Klara and Jonas a few steps away in the kitchen or talking in the living room didn't count. "Yeah, yeah," he would say with a knowing undertone in his voice, "you just play a tape with your voices on and then creep away secretly." Sometimes he even doubted whether Klara and Jonas were really themselves. Strangers could have disguised themselves as them and the real Klara and Jonas could be long gone. His suspicion was profound.

He was afraid that there was poison somewhere in his environment and found that his food tasted as if it were poisoned. Even before his father had left he had been careful with substances that seemed peculiar or smelt strange, like sap from trees, finger paints or sticky paper. When he came into contact with something like that, Adam had always washed his hands very carefully. But now he developed real paranoia. If he touched a foreign substance and then put his hands in his mouth by mistake, he would start to panic. He would cry and scream, his eyes wide with horror, asking if you could die from it. On holiday in Italy he tried five different kinds of water until he could finally accept one that didn't taste poisonous. And he continually washed his hands. Adam had lost faith in fundamental things: food, Mummy, Daddy, friends, playing, being happy.

It didn't do Adam's self-confidence any good either. The lack of sleep made him nervous and lacking in concentration. And then everything would go wrong: when he tried to whittle arrows like his dad had taught him, he cut his finger; when he wanted to make stars out of colored paper, they fell to pieces; when he wanted to make a house for Lilly's dolls out of bits of wood, everything collapsed and crushed his hand.

He stumbled from one catastrophe to the next. When he was drawing, the sketches went wrong right from the start and he lost all interest in the memory or board games that Lilly loved so much as soon as they were taken out of the box. Everything that he attempted went wrong. And he wasn't even surprised any more. It was quite clear to him: "I'm stupid." This became the stock phrase to be heard time and again.

For Adam everything made perfect sense: "Papa has left me because I'm so stupid." This was the explanation that he'd been looking for and that seemed logical to him. It could only be his fault and his alone that his father had gone away. Adam was quite sure of that. And his mother would also leave him because he was such a failure. Every evening he repeated these three things until he was exhausted: "I am frightened that you will go away; it's my fault that Papa has gone; I am stupid."

After a few weeks Adam looked as pale and transparent as a ghost and Klara was at her wits' end. They bought themselves a couple of nights' rest with a sedative from the doctor, but it was not a solution for his fear. Jonas knew a homeopath who had helped him greatly a while before. An attack of chronic gastritis had simply disappeared after taking a single dose of just five little globules. No more pain, no indigestion - he could eat normally again. For Jonas, a physicist by profession, it was pure magic and thus exactly what Adam needed now. Klara told the homeopath the whole story and as she showed him a photo in which Adam appeared thin and pale with deep dark rings under his eyes and with the belt around his chest to stop his heart from bursting, she fought back the tears.

The first separation from Ben had been traumatic for them all, explained Klara, because there had been absolutely no inkling that he was going to leave his family. It came completely out of the blue. In this respect she could understand his fear as something rational. Up until his sudden departure, Ben had always assured them that he loved them - just as Klara, Adam and Lilly loved him. One day he was there, then the next he was gone. But at that time Adam had not developed comparable panic attacks. He did suffer terribly, but he wasn't afraid.

Klara knows her son well and understands how he thinks. "He tries to solve all his problems using his head and that's why in his despair he has imagined the worst things that could possibly happen. At some level they were even very probable. It is plausible. I can tell him a hundred times: "You are the most important thing in the world for me, I'll never leave you, you're my life." But his father has told him that kind of thing too: "You're my one and only, you are my son" and hey presto, he has gone - twice. All things considered, his fear isn't exactly unfounded."

She can give exact descriptions of her son's behavioral patterns in his relationships with other children, with his father and with herself. "Adam can't cope with it when other boys keep fighting or playing the big man. Adam talks. He is a man of words and he wants to have discussions. He often pushes me to the limit of my ability to explain things. He wants to know things in detail and won't be put off with just any old answer. He wants to understand. And what happened with his father was just incomprehensible. Even now I can't understand it myself. I'm still looking for answers - but there just aren't any. How can you explain to a boy like him why his father deserted him? He needs his father. You can't explain it to him. Especially as they have such a close relationship. Ben loves his son and is really proud of him. Actually it really is impossible to understand."

Adam had never had much self-confidence even before this, says Klara. He has high expectations of himself which are not so easy to fulfill. When he does not live up to his expectations, he becomes impatient and thinks he's a total idiot again. But Adam doesn't only have high expectations of himself; it is extremely important for him that everyone obeys the rules. He takes it very seriously if someone fouls him or doesn't keep to what was agreed. It's the same if someone lies to him - that's a reason to stop being friends with them. In return, he is completely honest and reliable. This pattern can be seen in many areas of his life: Adam can't stand it if he sees that something is against the rules, if he is cheated of something or if he is in the right but the others are stronger than him.

Because of this he has huge problems with boys of his age. He gets on best with older girls. When he plays with them, things can be harmonious for days at a time.

When he was small, Adam was an open, jolly, sunny child, who began to speak early. Klara showed photos of a happy little boy who was obviously doing well. On one of the photos from his early years, a beaming child can be seen snuggling his head into the neck of his father, who is tenderly encircling his little son in his arms. As the first-born, Adam grew up primarily with adults to begin with. On the playground he watched his peers for a long time before joining in. Because he was naturally cautious, his way was to look first to see what was going on. That didn't change when he went to kindergarten. "He never liked going there," says Klara, although the carers all told her how wonderfully he fitted in and how popular he was and always in the thick of things. When he came home from kindergarten he was always in a terrible mood. He had to let all the pent-up aggression out at home. In kindergarten he appeared to keep himself under extremely tight control in order to appear uncomplicated to the others. Klara explains his behavior as wanting to appear to function well and fulfilling all demands perfectly.

But now nothing was functioning at all. He couldn't even get rid of his frustration - Adam was the stupidest idiot. He invested all his hope in the homeopathic globules. Klara reinforced this by promising that it was magic medicine. In a solemn ritual she laid the three globules on his tongue, kissed him goodnight and hoped for a miracle. But ten minutes later she was brought back to earth with a bump. Adam was sitting up in bed crying and screaming with fury, "Tell the doctor his magic pills are no good! I'm scared, I'm scared, I'm scared!" Subsequent nights continued as usual and the miracle failed to materialize even when Klara had given him the remedy a second time. At first Klara thought that this first medicine had not worked at all.

In retrospect, it was apparent that Adam had come a little nearer to the root of his problem. For the very first time he was able to express his fury and disappointment.

He dictated emails to his father which Klara typed into the computer word for word. For the first time he started to be angry with Ben and to let his frustration out. Now it was "stupid Daddy" not "darling Daddy." "Stupid Daddy," wrote Adam, "I am cross with you. Don't bother to come back - you are a stupid idiot." But at the same time he lay in bed every night crying and sobbing: "It's my fault and I love him. I want him to like me and he doesn't." However, Adam carried on with the emails. One was a favorite: "I am cross that you have gone. You are stupid, your children were cleverer - they told you to stay, but you went. Bye stupid daddy, I never want to see you again." Klara can't remember how many emails he sent, but it was a lot. Adam had dictated them with tears in his eyes. Klara knew that it was therapeutic for him - and for herself - to formulate his anger, but she saw that underlying it there was desperation and the feeling that he was not good enough to keep his father from leaving.

Perhaps this development was a step forward, a first step on the road to cure. But Adam's neurotic behavior didn't change. Still the same fight against going to sleep at night and by day, the same panic if he lost sight of his mother. She wasn't able to go to the toilet alone or disappear around a corner for a split second in the garden. And then there was the compulsive behavior. As well as the hand washing, there was the fight over his underpants. It started off with none of them being right, even though Klara had bought all the different kinds she could find and in different sizes. It took a while before he could finally decide on one and then there were temper tantrums because they pinched or didn't fit. He stood there every morning like Rumpelstiltskin, plucking at his pants and yelling, "I'm going to cut them up!" until Klara or Jonas shouted at him that he should keep his damned pants on. It might be OK for one day and then the fight would start again the next morning.

Adam was due to start school in a few months - unthinkable in the current situation. Klara wanted to try homeopathy again. Her homeopath chose a new remedy, closely related to the previous one and Klara administered the remedy with considerably less euphoria. Adam didn't have much faith in the supposedly magic globules, but allowed himself to be persuaded to take them. After a few minutes he went to sleep - with no problems and straight after the first dose. Just like that. Klara was so dumbfounded that she wrote her homeopath the following email: "It is probably still too early to celebrate, but last night gives me hope." This time the hope was justified. From then on Adam slept peacefully as if there had never been a problem. The nightmare was over, gone as quickly as it had come. For a few weeks he was haunted by a new fear - that certain strange-looking women were witches. As far as Klara was concerned, it was a fair exchange. This fear was not unusual for a six-year-old and he was easily reassured. The fear of witches soon dissipated without any more magic pills.

Adam still goes to sleep well and sleeps through the night. His compulsive hand-washing has gone. He is still occasionally troubled by a fear of being poisoned, but not particularly seriously. He has become a bit braver in general and goes to school by bus and does gymnastics and football. The best thing is that he likes it. When the homeopath asks what has happened to his fear he answers, "I've put it in a box." And what about the voices on the tapes and the strangers who dressed up as Mummy and Jonas while the real ones ran away? "That's a silly question - I know that they're not going anywhere!" he says in a tone of voice that shows he is absolutely certain of it.

Commentary

Critics of homeopathy like to explain the success of the therapy with the placebo effect. This is an effect which is not due to the medicine itself but to the personality and attention of the practitioner, reinforced by the trust of the patient and his belief in the healing powers of the remedy. According to scientific findings the placebo effect, closely related to the theory of spontaneous healing, plays a greater or lesser role in all forms of medicine, from shamanic healing ritual through to heart by-pass surgery and chemotherapy. However, according to critics of homeopathy, the placebo effect is solely responsible for its success. In Adam's case, the conditions for a magical placebo phenomenon were optimal. Homeopathy had already been proved to the family to be a particularly effective method of healing. Knowing this, Adam had great faith in the magic globules. But neither the belief in it nor the ritual of taking it helped the homeopathic remedy achieve its desired aim. Adam made no secret of his disappointment. Those so-called wonder pills were just no good.

That was the starting point for the second try with homeopathy. The globules had been thoroughly demystified and Adam, by nature suspicious, couldn't have had an ounce of faith in them. In such a situation one would assume that a negative placebo effect would take place, whereby the efficacy of the remedy is hindered rather than reinforced by the attitude and expectations of the patient. Accordingly, it was a huge surprise when Adam went to sleep a few minutes after taking the second remedy. It was as if someone had pressed a button and simply switched the fear off. Suddenly Adam was sleeping normally again although nothing in his external situation had changed.

Adam's reaction to the separation of his parents was not unusual - it was in many ways even typical for children of divorced parents in his age-group. The break-up of a family throws any child – shakes their trust in their parents and causes fear of abandonment. Loss of security also affects the child's sense of self which is dependent on the parents to a high degree. As in Adam's case, pronounced feelings of inferiority often arise out of this situation. These feelings allow children to conclude that they are the reason for the inexplicable behavior of their parents. Particularly at the ages of six and below, children typically consider themselves to be the reason for the withdrawal of love. That is why Daddy can only have gone away because Adam is a stupid idiot. That is the most logical conclusion according to Adam's view of the world.

The homeopath must then judge to what degree Adam's reaction exceeds the usual level of uncertainty experienced by children in a divorce situation. What is unusual and individual in his psychological symptoms?

To begin with, the intensity of his fear and suspicion is striking. This means he needs a homeopathic remedy which would cause similarly existential fear and similarly great suspicion in a healthy person. What distinguishes Adam from other children in a similar situation and is particularly striking is his strange fear of being poisoned. This fear of poisoning must be in the remedy picture of his simillimum, as must the main problem, sleeplessness due to fear. This symptom is found in the rubric "Sleeplessness – fear, from" in the repertory. The characteristics of Adam's unhealthy mental state point to one particular substance that was formerly used to poison rats - and sometimes humans: arsenic, of all things. Central to the remedy picture of *Arsenicum album*, white oxide of arsenic or arsenous acid, are harrowing fears and pronounced paranoia.

Arsenicum album is one of a whole family of chemically related homeopathic remedies containing arsenic (see also the Glossary showing the periodic table). Symptoms of fear and paranoia typical for the arsenic content are common to them all. The additional component in the chemical compound adds extra aspects to the remedy picture. This principle is founded on the hypothesis of the much-quoted Dutch chemist and homeopath Jan Scholten. According to Scholten, the remedy pictures of compounds such as salts or acids consist of a combination of the themes and characteristics of the constituent elements. Numerous remedy pictures constructed in this way for the many compound remedies in the group have been confirmed in clinical practice.

Adam was able to profit from Scholten's theory, but not at the first attempt. Initially the homeopath made the wrong combination. He had given him *Calcarea arsenicosa*, the calcium salt of arsenous acid. The calcium content represents the themes of safety and security, which in the salt combine with the keynotes of suspicion and fear of arsenicum. The essence of the remedy is thus insecurity and harrowing fear because one cannot trust the people on whom one's safety and security depend. This picture of *Calcarea arsenicosa* seems to represent the crux of Adam's problem. However, the remedy did not work. As the little patient pointed out - the granules were just no good.

But the remedy was close to the simillimum. The next remedy given was another salt of arsenic. There was no doubt as to the patient's panic and paranoia, but what was the cause of his profound suspicion? It wasn't so much about a safe and secure home as in the calcium salts, but rather it was the fear that the people closest to him would deceive and abandon him - a fear based on painful experience. Taking this into consideration, the remedy *Natrium arsenicosum* was prescribed. The natrium part in a compound generally represents a disturbance in the relationship to loved-ones, usually caused by a loss or a great disappointment. Thus *Natrium arsenicosum* covers the crux of Adam's problem even more exactly than *Calcarea arsenicosa*. In addition, the homeopathic repertory offers further symptoms for this salt that correspond closely with his state of mind. We find the "delusion he is worthless" which coincides with Adam's feeling of being "a stupid idiot" and also the rubric "Reproaches himself" which equates exactly with Adam's feelings of guilt. "Fear at night in bed" also typifies the homeopathic remedy picture for *Natrium arsenicosum*. This remedy reflects the major characteristics of the unusual condition into which Adam slipped after the second separation from his father and thus holds the vital impetus which the organism needs to restore its balance.

In the remedy *Calcarea arsenicosa*, the themes of inferiority and guilt which were so marked in Adam are missing. This remedy does not match the disease picture accurately enough to bring about a complete cure according to the Law of Similars. Even ideal conditions for the placebo effect couldn't compensate for this lack. This corresponds with daily experience in homeopathic practice. The first remedy given does not always lead to success. Adam's completely different reaction to the first and second remedies is not only interesting in relation to the placebo discussion - it also shows how precisely homeopathic remedies must be prescribed.

12. The Prince in the Caul or The Child of Fortune

> *The unconscious world of mythological symbols speaks indirectly to that which is ruled by the external world through the experience of external things. In the same way, the real external world and its demands speak indirectly to that which is ruled purely by the soul. This is because no one can escape the two realities.*
>
> *If a person concentrates solely on the external world, he must live his myth and if he concentrates solely on his inner life, he must dream his external so-called real life.*
>
> C.G. Jung

Once upon a time there was a young king who loved the beauty of nature above all things and much preferred playing his violin in the forest to ruling his kingdom. He was at home in the realms of myth and the soul, not in the workshops of reason or the forges of order in the external world. He could not speak the language of the bold men of action from whom he was descended and he did not want to. The political business of the world bored him to the extreme. Let the young queen take on his duties as well as she could, he thought - he didn't mind. She was a child of the fairy world and had renounced her people out of love for the king. She was certainly not born to rule the world of man and everyone in the nation knew where she came from. Her long golden-red curls reached to her feet, glowing like maple leaves in the autumn forest. Her voice sounded like the tinkling bubble of mountain springs and her robes were made of poppy flowers and maidenhair ferns.

The king and queen had seven daughters who were as daring and bold as imps. They would much rather go out hunting than learn the customs and traditions of court, even though the queen was tirelessly concerned about their education. The king's council came together and told the king, "Lord, your daughters are as daring and bold as imps, but they will not be suitable for ruling the country. The kingdom needs a hand that will keep it in order. You know, Lord, what the situation is. The Iron King of the Land of Ores is threatening to levy troops and to overrun us if we don't open ourselves to the New World and become a match for the men of action. Queen Tabea, Queen of Fairyland and mother of your consort, has also counseled that we need to build a bridge between the Old and the New Worlds. Because, Lord, we need both beauty and order."

"O noble council," sighed the king, "what shall I do?" The old Master of Ceremonies whispered something in his ear. The king went a little red, said nothing and stopped sighing. He did not play his violin for a while either. In the course of the year a child was born. The king and queen were beside themselves with joy because it was a little boy, born enveloped in a miraculous shimmering lucky skin. The news spread quickly throughout the world "A son is born in the Middle Kingdom - an heir who came into the world safe in a lucky skin." The whole nation pinned their hopes on the Child of Fortune who would one day surely succeed in building the bridge between the worlds, once he was mature and grown and sitting on the throne. The magic of the lucky skin even touched the Iron King of the Land of Ores and he swore to the high council and the government that he would keep the peace for a while longer.

The king and queen believed in their Child of Fortune even more than anyone else and trusted that everything would take its course, so they carried on as before. The high councilors nodded their heads thoughtfully; the young king praised the beauty of Nature and played his violin enchantingly; and the young queen wove herself new clothes from peach blossom and ivy tendrils and tried to control her seven wild daughters who still preferred going out hunting rather than learning the customs and traditions of court.

It did not trouble the king and queen that their Child of Fortune did not want to speak, even though he was over three years old. "Oh," thought the young queen when her dumb son smiled at her, "the Child of Fortune will find the right words one day - there's no hurry. Fate must mean well by a prince who is born in a lucky skin." And without delay she wrapped the little one in her blossomy robes, tied him onto her back and chased after her wild daughters once more, to keep them from the worst.

One day she was resting, exhausted, in a forest glade and fell asleep. The Child of Fortune got off her back and snuggled deeply into the moss to dream. The queen awoke to the noise of her seven daughters who were dancing around her in a tight circle; they caught her up in their wild round dance and roared through the forest with her like a storm. Their boisterous play did not finish until they were back at the castle and the queen sank onto her bed out of breath. It was long after nightfall when she realized that the cradle was empty. The queen was shocked to the core and terrified lest something should have happened to the Child of Fortune in the forest.

Just as the queen felt this fear, a strange man stepped out of the wall of her quarters. He was wrapped in a dark blue cloak in which all the colors of the sea were woven and he handed her the little sleeping prince, who soon awoke and looked around in astonishment.

"My Lady," he said, "I counsel you to look out for this Child of Fortune. His lucky skin alone will not protect him. And," he continued, "take heed of the games your daughters play. They think it is good sport to tease the prince until he cries - and they don't stop there. They revel in his sorrow and say, 'So you want to be a Child of Fortune, you poor little worm! You can't even speak. And you can't stand up for yourself. How are you going to keep up with us? And how are you ever going to rule our kingdom?'"

The queen answered, "My seven daughters surely wish their brother no ill - they have just invented a new game that they are enjoying." "You are mistaken, O Queen," said the magician. "They have realized what you do not wish to see. They are playing the game of the strong and your Child of Fortune is weak. The magic of the lucky skin alone will not help the little prince if he wishes to succeed in life. But I want to help you." He opened his fist and offered her a bowl which shimmered in all the colors of the sea. "Look inside," he said, "and you will see that I am right." The queen looked into the bowl as into a mirror and asked the Child of Fortune a question. The Child of Fortune answered with strange sounds, as was his wont. The noises he made sounded like the bubbling of a mountain spring or the rustling of a lime green forest in spring. Instead of words, a few tiny pebbles actually tumbled out of his mouth. The queen thanked the stranger and promised him to look after the Child of Fortune better.

Now they recognized that their son was not able to form even the simplest word correctly. The queen soon ordered that the child be taught by a private tutor and the most senior lady-in-waiting. But the Child of Fortune did not want to learn. He wanted to carry on dreaming in his own little world and stay safe inside his own skin and not go out to the others. His big dark eyes said, "Leave me in my hidey-hole, Mother." The queen held the prince's head in her hands, gently kissed his lips and promised to protect him for ever; he could always stay with her and would never have to go out into the world. She wanted to forget the magician.

So everything took its course and everyone carried on as usual. The high council nodded their heads even more thoughtfully; the young king sang the praises of nature even more highly and played his violin better and better. The young queen made new dresses out of white camellias and tender palm leaves, watched over the little prince and tried with all her might to tame her wild daughters, who would still much rather go out hunting than learn the customs and traditions of court. But the Child of Fortune withdrew further and further into his dream world and sometimes, when the queen remembered the shimmering bowl and the strange man, a tiny tear trickled down her cheek. For sometimes, as if in a vague fog, she had an inkling that the Child of Fortune, who still couldn't speak, would never sit on the throne and rule the land if something didn't change. For who would respect a dumb king?

The years passed by until finally the Iron King of the Land of Ores amassed his troops at the borders of the land, as he had threatened to do before. According to the news that reached him, there was little prospect of the Child of Fortune keeping his side of the bargain. When the king heard this he was so worried that he forgot his violin and asked the high council what was to be done. But they just shook their heads. Even the old Master of Ceremonies didn't know what to do. The queen got out the shimmering bowl, took a long look into it and cried a tiny, very beautiful, perfect pearl. Then she immediately left her seven bold daughters to their wild games and wrapped the Child of Fortune in her flowery robes, tied him to her back and went to the glade in the forest where she had once left him. Just as she had ardently wished, the magician was standing in the middle of the glade, which was flooded with the light of the full moon.

In his hands he held a bowl that shimmered with all the colors of the seas and the waters - just like the first bowl, but larger and more magnificent. "O my Lady," sighed the magician, "you have not heeded my advice, but I will still help you. I will ask the Iron King of the Land of Ores to delay a little longer if you will finally start to fight and help your child to gain the confidence to take his first steps alone into the world. Let him walk around the glade, look into the mirror bowl and you will see what to do. Looking in the mirror, the queen saw what she had not been able or willing to see before. Her little prince walked so slowly that the seasons changed quicker than his steps. And for the first time she noticed how badly he limped and how he suffered great pain when he dragged his left leg.

Thereupon, the king and queen and the high council summoned all the wise men and women and healers from throughout the world to help the Child of Fortune. Medicine men also came from the New World. They looked through the Child of Fortune's bones with their magic metal mirrors and found that in the royal hip, the seat of the pain, where it was at its hottest and burned like fire, there was something sealed in and encapsulated. It was in the head of the femur, they pronounced wisely, and perhaps 'it' would disappear in time or break out once and for all and destroy the bone completely. Then they pointed to their scalpels and instruments and offered to cut out from the head of the femur the sealed-in and encapsulated 'thing' and get rid of it.

But the queen feared for the life of her little prince and fell into deep despair. She cried a whole soup-bowlful of her beautiful, tiny, perfect pearls and cradled her child in her arms day and night. She could see that he was no longer eating and sleeping and that his big dark eyes were full of pain. And to her horror, she also saw that the little stones held in his mouth instead of words had by no means gone, but had become bigger and were stuck even more firmly in his teeth and must hurt and burn like the fire that lit the castle by night. She feared no one could save her son. Without even wrapping her child in her flowery robes and binding him to her back as she usually did, she carried him in her outstretched arms and flew, her golden-red mane flowing behind her, to the clearing where the magician was already waiting for her.

"O my Lady!" he said and sighed deeply three times. "Do you not know who sent me to you? It was Tabea your mother, full of sympathy for you. Why have you and your consort not taken her advice to heart and carried out the task you were given, to build a bridge between the Old World and the New? Your heir, the Child of Fortune, dumb and weak as he is, will not be able to do it. Do you really believe that anything will happen without your taking a hand in the matter? Tabea wanted to help you and your seven daughters and above all the little prince. That's why she sent me and the bowls that shimmer in all the colors of the seas and the waters. Do you not recognize the value of these gifts? Why are your tears like tiny pearls? It is a medicine that will make the Child of Fortune healthy and strong."

And he gave the queen another bowl like the others but even more magnificent, that sparkled in all the colors of the seas and the stars. So smooth, so perfect, so beautiful. Inside, the queen saw encompassed by the concentric rings of the bowl, a pearl that glittered and shone with all the colors of the rainbow, like a dewdrop from heaven or a tear from the Gods.

"Mother of pearl. That is the medicine that your mother Tabea sent you. Now O Queen, listen well and shave off a few grains of mother of pearl and grind it together with milk sugar again and again all night long and give the powder to the child. And then you will see what happens." As the queen, crying pearly tears of joy, gave her hand to the magician to thank him, he transformed himself into a being that was like her mother, the Queen of Fairyland and somehow like all mothers and fathers she had ever seen in her life. The long white hair surrounded the form of the being like a glacier that never melts, but the farewell blessing sounded as warm as a summer breeze tumbling down from the mountains. It was like the wings of wild geese that fly to the south only to return, and like the endless waves of the ocean that enfold the land in the eternal ebb and flow of the tides.

Then the young queen understood and gave her child the medicine. Three months later the seven daughters stopped teasing the Child of Fortune, because he didn't cry any more. He left his sisters to their wild hunting and games and devoted himself to growing and to knowledge. The stones in his mouth disappeared, as did his pain. And then came the words. At first only letters and syllables surfaced, but then longer and longer words followed by simple sentences. Then sentences with comical interjections and fancy endings thrust themselves out of his mouth - and there was always laughter between all the clever things that the child suddenly knew. Before all this, the burning pain in the head of his femur and in his joints had stopped and the prince stopped limping. His stride was perhaps not as bold as that of his sisters - but quite in keeping with most other children. And so he dared to take his first steps out into the world and became braver and bolder until at last he could pursue ever higher and more distant goals in his young life.

When the Child of Fortune had grown into a mature young man, he built under the benevolent eyes of his father and the pacified Iron King of the Land of Ores a wonderfully curved and extremely durable bridge between the Old World and the New. And so he united beauty and order. The world of the childlike soul and holy myths was now connected to the world of the workshops and forges where was done what had to be done. So from that time on, anyone could move between the worlds whenever he pleased. And so the Child of Fortune became mature and intelligent in readiness for the throne of the Middle Kingdom and he, the king and queen and their seven daughters (who remained as bold and daring as imps) all lived joyfully and with the blessing of their people until the end of their days.

Commentary:

There really is a prince in a lucky skin. In the eyes of his mother at least, Felix is a prince, even if he will not inherit a kingdom. He was indeed born in a caul, the intact amniotic sac that shimmers at birth like mother of pearl. From time immemorial this has been called a lucky skin and has been seen as a good omen for the life of the child. This is the case, for example, in the fairy tale "The Devil and the Three Golden Hairs." In this story the princess is the lucky child's prize, but first he must complete three difficult tasks, through which he can mature and grow. Development and growth are issues for Felix, which is why we have told his story as a fairy tale. This is the classical literary form concerning individuation, the development of the personality and the task of carving out one's place in the world. This process isn't really getting off the ground with Felix.

Felix's mother and father are both emotional, musical and concerned for the environment. They believe in allowing their children to develop naturally without external pressure to achieve. With their loving way of dealing with their children, they do not want to regulate either the strong personalities of their two daughters or the shy withdrawal of their son. Because they believe humankind to be naturally part of a harmonious whole, they trust that their little boy, their third child, will progress naturally - even though he seems a bit slow and backward and finds it difficult to speak. The parents see the superior strength of his two older sisters as the reason why Felix refuses to conquer the world. They want to give him time, and don't press him - perhaps they are in denial a little bit. Felix learns to speak late and slowly and even then he stutters. He is backward in everything, doesn't want to learn, is often unmanageable and totally in his own world. And he remains in the shadow of his two older, very dominant sisters, unable to stand up to them. Somehow he always seems to be limping along behind.

At five he does begin to limp due to a painful disease of the hips called Legg-Calvé-Perthes disease, which gives the clear signal that Felix needs help. This circulatory disturbance of the head of the femur, not that unusual in boys of his age, is actually a boon for Felix because it shows the way to a remedy that will not only fix his hip, but will also set his whole faltering development in motion. As in our fairy tale, Felix is given 'Mater Perlarum', ground mother of pearl from the inside of an oyster shell.

The homeopathic usage of mother of pearl dust goes back to observations in the nineteenth century. Austrian doctors noticed that primarily young employees in mother of pearl workshops often developed strange inflammations of the heads of their long bones. The disease could begin suddenly with fever and bone pains near a joint that would quickly stop on immobilization. Some workers got the same illness again if they stayed in their jobs. This is the toxological background to the homeopathic prescription of mother of pearl in a case of Legg-Calvé-Perthes disease. According to the Law of Similars, *Conchiolinum* (the remedy made from mother of pearl), can help the kind of bone complaints that the substance caused in the mother of pearl cutters.

However, the experienced homeopath who prescribed *Conchiolinum* for Felix had further reasons for choosing this remedy. She sees a correlation between the acute disease picture, the personal development of the boy and the origin of the remedy. The part stands for the whole: the local symptom in the hips embodies a fundamental problem in his personality, which in turn finds a similarity in the picture of the seashell. Felix is as stuck as a pearl in an oyster and is out of touch with his environment. It is as if he is still in his caul - his lucky skin - and is cut off from the world. In the worst case, the encapsulated disease process in his hips could lead to necrosis and the death of bone tissue, which would prevent him stepping out into the world for a very long time. In this way Felix's body expresses his internal distress physically and directs the homeopath's attention to his retarded development.

Conchiolinum is not one of the remedies well known for this problem. Not much is known about the remedy and in the past it was only prescribed for the bone disorder and respiratory problems common as occupational diseases in mother of pearl cutters. One of the classical homeopathic remedies for arrested childhood development, especially in speech, is *Calcarea carbonica.* This is not just any old preparation of calcium - according to Hahnemann's directions, it is made from the ground-up middle layer of an oyster shell. This remedy thus comes from the same source as *Conchiolinum*; mother of pearl however, is the inner layer of the oyster shell and it contains proteins as well as calcium. According to the aforementioned method of group analysis, the similarity of origin between *Calcarea carbonica* and *Conchiolinum* would lead us to expect a comparable homeopathic sphere of action and thus we can expect that potentised mother of pearl can influence arrested childhood development in the same way as calcium carbonate from the oyster shell.

Felix's reaction to taking the homeopathic remedy made from mother of pearl dust confirms the assumption. To start with, the hip pains disappear overnight. Later, *Conchiolinum* helps just as quickly with inflammation in a filled tooth - another problem in an enclosed capsule. Felix used to suffer extremely badly from caries in his milk teeth - the stones in our fairy tale. The main progress, however, occurs on another level. The shell opens, Felix makes contact and speaks. All at once his speech becomes differentiated; he uses complicated grammatical constructions and special vocabulary. He has opinions about things and comes out of himself. His mother says, "Now he actively takes part in conversations, which he never did before." And he defends himself against his older sisters. Before, he would burst out crying when they taunted him with a prized toy that they would keep taking away from him. Now he carries on with what he is doing and says, "You won't give it to me anyway."

If you meet the seven-year-old Felix today, he is a lively lad, linguistically talented and communicative, even with people he doesn't know. He takes them into his room, shows them his drawings and goes on about his shiny silver cars. Two years after treatment his parents remember his physical illness clearly, but hardly remember the delay in his development. So distant, indeed, are his mother's memories of her prince's former weakness that she worries instead about his recent aggressive behavior. Like other boys of his age, he is now starting to fight. In the playground he even scraps with his sisters when their attacks get too much for him. Felix's mother is very surprised that their once so gentle boy defends himself so vehemently. Now it's no problem for him to stay at home alone with his sisters - an amazing novelty for his mother after the remedy. He is no longer afraid and feels safe. He now goes skiing and doesn't hold back from steeper slopes. Furthermore he has started to learn a musical instrument and is very focused on it. His mother summarizes his development since taking the remedy *Conchiolinum* two years ago in one sentence: "His old clothes don't fit him any more."

Unlike in the story of Maria in the second chapter, there is no serious retardation or deep-seated constitutional problem in this case. Felix would have eventually made his way even without homeopathic treatment. However, this example shows how a person's development can be given a boost with a well-chosen homeopathic remedy. It is as if a blockage is released. The person can access his vitality and his inner resources better. In this way - as shown in most of our stories - the remedy contribute to individualization. The fairy tale of the Prince in the Caul symbolizes this important aspect of the homeopathic healing process.

13. If the Ice Breaks…

Man becomes ill because he never comes to rest.
Paracelsus

Grete had a dream. Every year, when the crisp cold came and strange frost patterns formed on the windows, the dream came - every night. "Pack your bags, quick, quick. Just take what you need - don't forget anything. We've got to go. Out into the cold, out onto the ice." Then she woke up bathed in sweat, terrified. Thank God, only a dream. But the fear stayed with her all day, went to her stomach and robbed her of her peace of mind. It had been happening for most of her life now.

She would need days to recount it all, to tell us about her life, about what made her ill and what made her healthy. "Oh dear," says Grete and sighs and smiles. But it's this one night she speaks about again and again. The memory of it, the darkness, the terror, the noises, the fear of the next moment. And again she says, "Oh dear, if I were to tell you….. it'd take days." Then she pauses. She is upset, very upset. Even now her heart beats like mad when she has to speak about "that." Actually she wanted to talk about the homeopathic remedy that helped her so much, but instead she is talking about her theme - flight. She still hasn't got over it, she says. But how can you assimilate mortal fear? Even though you've had a lifetime to do it like Grete?

The Vistula Lagoon - it was there they had to cross the ice. There was no other way - East Prussia was cut off in January 1945, surrounded by the Red Army. The eastern front held by the Central German Army Group had collapsed the summer before. Senior generals urged that the population be evacuated. Hitler refused. The powers that be ordered that any escape attempt be severely punished.

Both Grete's older brothers were at the front or in Königsberg (Kaliningrad) - where exactly they didn't know. The Russians had already entered East Prussia. At first they heard on the radio that the remaining German soldiers had held them off, but then the Russians advanced and stormed forwards, unstoppable. Only a few places had any defences, amongst them Heiligenbeil, Grete's home town. It was there that her parents' house stood with its garden, where she had her roots as a child.

The Red Army was soon so close that you could hear the dull rumble of the artillery and the tanks. The howls of the multiple rocket launchers with their volleys of missiles were terrifying. A few days or maybe only a few hours and they would be here.

The Vistula Spit, a narrow strip of land to the south west of Königsberg, was the only escape route to Danzig (Gdansk) and further west. To get to it, they had to cross the frozen lagoon of the Baltic Sea. It was minus $20\,^{\circ}C$ on those ice-cold January days. The icy sludge had begun to freeze into ice floes that bumped and rubbed against each other in the persistent cold, growing into huge pancakes of ice with turned-up edges that joined to form an uneven surface. The cracked carpet of ice reached to the strip of land. The ice seemed to be firm, but would it carry all those people? There would be more than two million people wanting to cross the lagoon to reach either the safety of dry land or the refugee ships out in the Baltic.

Grete's father was still not allowed to leave in January 1945; he had to stay at his post guarding the airfield at Heiligenbeil - even when everyone knew that it was hopeless. If he had left, he would have been shot. So the twelve-year-old girl had to leave with her mother and her eldest brother's wife with their seven-month-old child. Grete tries to smile. "We managed it in half an hour - we already had our air-raid bags ready, because of the low-flying aircraft. You must remember I was a child - I stood in front of our canary and wanted to take it with us - I remember that to this day. And then we crossed the lagoon with my sister-in-law and the baby." The lagoon - always the lagoon.

Grete didn't understand why they had to leave. Nobody, least of all her parents, had told the sheltered baby of the family the horror stories which spread like wildfire before the advancing Russian troops, fanned by Nazi propaganda. The adults knew about the bloody brutalities, the terror and brutal plundering, the mass rape of women and children. Grete knew nothing about all that. She just felt dragged away, torn out of her house and garden in Heiligenbeil.

The construction of the Ostwall (East Wall) defenses and slogans about ultimate victory had given the population a false sense of security, so most people didn't leave until the front was within earshot. The Great Trek in the bitter cold in overloaded carts or on foot became the Great Death. Thousands were left behind; some froze, others were blown to pieces by bombs, fell through the ice of the Vistula Lagoon or died of exhaustion. Many were caught by the Soviet tanks and crushed to death, victims of the hatred sown by Germans before them.

Later, while Grete was on her month-long flight with its many ports of call, she got to know a young girl, only a little older than herself, who died from her wounds. The grown-ups only talked in whispers about her because some of "them" had "done something to her." Grete didn't understand, but what she felt was the fear. The fear of her mother, who had survived the First World War, the fear of her young sister-in-law and the quaking fear of her father who was a weak man - too weak to give his family hope.

Grete remembers the last meal at home. It was early afternoon and there was soup with winter vegetables. The White Russians, prisoners of war, sat with them at the table. They were not meant to give them anything to eat, but Grete's mother was a Christian woman. It was a meager but warming meal, and then they left. It was a grey day and already getting dark, perhaps between three and four when they joined the trek. The streets were full of women and children and old people who pushed and shoved and tried to get the overloaded carts going. "You can't imagine what it was like - everywhere was blocked. People were unloading what they'd just loaded so they just had a little suitcase - the horses couldn't carry it all - but then we were on the water - not on the water, on the ice - that was the worst..." It is so bad that Grete can only tell us in fragments and broken sentences. She knows that they went on foot and then for a while on a wagon. "No, not a sled that could have slid across the ice - it was wagons with wheels that cut into the frozen water.

We heard the glugging on all sides. It was dark - you could only cross in the dark or they'd have shot you…. Anything that was still there - horses and carts, hand carts and trailers - everything had to be used to save people. They couldn't go to and fro - that wasn't possible. The lagoon was twelve kilometers wide. But I don't know how long it took us - I don't know, it was dark - had to be dark - the low-flying aircraft - it cracked to the left and to the right and then you heard cries for help and the 'glug glug' as they sank..." No, Grete could not tell us any more graphically.

Grete was surrounded by groaning, bursting, cracking ice. What she heard was a dark rumbling and roaring in the depths which continued further and further underneath and what she experienced was the clinking and cracking on the surface. The ice could not hold the multitude of people. The crystal carpet began to tear in all directions. Unpredictable in the darkness of the night but undeniably near - everywhere. Would the splitting and cracking force its way to her feet? Would Grete sink into the icy waters of the Baltic - like the others sinking all around her with their horses and carts, mothers, siblings, grandparents? The gurgling and screaming didn't last long. But still every time it seemed to last an eternity. When would it get her or her mother or her sister-in-law with the baby on the wagon? Grete stepped over bundles out of which little faces stared. Babies and toddlers that had frozen to death and had been left behind on the ice by their mothers. Any second of this trip, which seemed to Grete to last an eternity, the ice could give beneath her and with her next step a gaping crack between the ice floes could swallow her up. Twelve kilometers of it - twelve thousand meters. Someone always went ahead, prodded and knocked with a big stick to see if the ice would hold, then turned around, waved and called, "Come on." On and on. Grete's mother sat silent and stiff on the wagon with her hands folded in prayer. Who by God's Will would sink and who would not? To this day Grete believes that if you can't live by the Will of God, you can't live at all. Your fate is determined. Even the worst thing in her life - the Lagoon.

Grete crossed the ice. In the gray of early morning she felt firm land underfoot. But it would be decades before she could put down roots again. They continued on foot and by horse and cart. The passenger steamer "Wilhelm Gustloff" was waiting for the refugees at Danzig. "Thank God we didn't get on the ship," says Grete. "We were lucky." On May 30th 1945 the "Gustloff" weighed anchor in the Bay of Danzig. No one on board could know that a soviet submarine was following the ocean giant. As night fell, three torpedoes tore into the "Gustloff". She sank only sixty minutes later and over nine thousand refugees died. Grete is still filled with disbelief when she talks about it. "A tragedy - the few children who survived had no relatives left."

The fear of losing her mother on the journey west is as unforgettable for Grete as the night on the lagoon. They had to cross the river Weichsel. All the bridges had been destroyed and there was hopeless chaos as thousands of people vied to get taken over the river first. Suddenly her mother was gone - submerged in the mass of people, not to be found. Grete ran to and fro, the panic rising in her. "The most beautiful slap in the face of my life" brought Grete back to earth. Out of shock, her mother had clouted her little daughter when she saw her emerge from the mass of people. They lost each other again at a station but found each other again at their destination, Regenwalde. Grete had already settled down there as best she could, but her mother drove her on. Once again it was: "Pack your bags, quick, we must go. Get on the train, all aboard!" The train stopped after a few kilometers on an open piece of track. As they looked back, they could see that Regenwalde was ablaze. The Russians. They had been lucky again.

Somewhere near Bremerhaven they could get no further west. The refugees stayed there, unwelcome scroungers, tolerated at best. They lived here and there with farmers who were obliged to take the refugees in. They got food for work and, like the other refugee children, Grete didn't go to school for years. In all the villages animals were slaughtered illicitly. The farmers had enough to eat. And then came Grete, thin and hungry - a "refugee lass" as the north Germans called her. "Yes," they said once graciously, "you may sit at the table with us and eat." Grete felt humiliated and inferior, a feeling that she never forgot all her life. Maybe she was more sensitive than others - I still am today she explains. Being sensitive - to Grete that means being upset, being afraid and feeling panic when others remain completely relaxed.

When they finally found a place to stay, Grete became seriously ill with vomiting, weight loss, pains and weakness. A German military doctor diagnosed her through the barbed wire fence of a prison camp. "Why are you bringing this child to me? She's got hepatitis, can't you see that?" Grete's skin was as yellow as ripe quince and the doctor was afraid of being infected. He couldn't help - there was no medicine. So there remained only household remedies such as sheep's lice packed in plums to draw the poison out of Grete's body. After a six-week diet of curd cheese, Grete was still very weak, but no longer yellow. She recovered very slowly and only weighed thirty kilograms at the age of thirteen. The symptoms of being unable to eat properly without her stomach rebelling, bad liver function and a tendency to cramps and vomiting remained with her.

When she was nineteen, Grete fell in love with Alfred, a young refugee from West Prussia who was also nineteen. Grete's father, who had not found his family until years after the war, was against Alfred. His reaction was to berate his daughter: "What are you thinking? You have nothing and you are a nobody – just like him. What good can come of it?" But as Grete said, lightning had already struck. In 1951 a daughter was born and naturally they got married. The three of them lived in barracks in a refugee camp. Alfred was unemployed like the rest of them. There was seven Marks dole money and in order to get it and remain eligible for a pension, Grete had to plant young trees in the forest. Grete's illness flared up again after the birth of her daughter and she felt absolutely terrible with bad liver function, weakness and weight loss. But still she had to do heavy labor. For a while, a friend planted the trees for Grete as her condition was so wretched. Life in the barracks was hard. Alfred got up at four in the morning, fetched water in a bucket and boiled the nappies on the stove. He did everything so that Grete could feel a bit more comfortable. They endured it for two years.

When their son was on the way, Alfred decided to start a new life with his family in southern Germany. But Grete's father threatened, "If you take that child and go away, I'll hang myself!" so they took her parents with them and looked after them for twelve years until they died. "Nowadays they put people in homes," says Grete. But she never mentioned that to Alfred until forty-eight years later, a week before his death; it had never been an issue between them. "That's how we gave up a huge part of our youth. Today everyone lives their own life and the old people are shunted off. I don't know - perhaps I'd be selfish today too." There is no trace of bitterness in her voice; it's more guilt, because Alfred's answer to her doubts was simple: "Selfish? Not me!"

Meeting Alfred was a stroke of luck for Grete. If her husband had not supported her as he did all through their life together and if he had not always tried to keep at bay everything that frightened her, she would not have been able to live with these things. Things which pursued her in her dreams at night and left her no peace during the day. Her neck trembled with agitation. She was frantic and driven by fear. Fear of everyone and everything. Fear for the children, in case anything happened to them, in case they didn't come home from school. Fear when they went on journeys, fear of change, fear of every step into the future. The fear didn't release its hold in her new life either. It made repeated inroads into her body with stomach cramps, vomiting and weakness - even when, thanks to her energetic husband, they were well provided for in their new life, the children were grown up and independent and she and her husband had long since retired. Then Alfred had his first stroke and Grete became very ill.

The GP diagnosed gastritis and treated her with antibiotics. Everything became worse. There was only one medicine that helped and that grew in her garden. At some point she had noticed that her stomach complaints got better if she ate salsify. At times the white roots with the sticky black skin became her staple diet. "I could live on it," she told Dr. Welte, the homeopath her daughter sent her to. He decided to conduct an experiment. A few fresh roots from Grete's garden were washed, ground in a porcelain pot, preserved in alcohol for three weeks and then potentised as directed in the homeopathic pharmacopeia. In this manner, *Scorzonera* 30 C was made, a remedy that was otherwise unavailable at that time.

One week after taking the potentised salsify, Grete is practically symptom free. She can eat everything again and keep the food down without her stomach complaining. The serious intestinal inflammation that had been made worse by the antibiotics improves and her bowel movements also become normal again. After two months she starts to put on weight for the first time in a long while. Later Grete realizes that some things have changed fundamentally - and not just her stomach. She is not a scientist and has not been to university, but one thing she does understand: body and soul are connected.

Grete describes her new lease of life: "It is as if peace has come, when you can compose yourself, when you can become quiet again." She has become more balanced with this remedy, which she calls her "wonder remedy." She knows that the agitation and the fears didn't come from her childhood; she wasn't born with them. She wasn't like that as a child - she was protected. Everything came afterwards, after the flight. Now all the fears that have accompanied her throughout her life have gone. She is no longer afraid of the future and is not afraid of getting old or of pain. She has also lost her fear of humiliation and being inferior and her fear of dreams - she does not have to pack her bags and go any more. She has found her inner peace. Everyone around her notices how her agitation and frantic activity have lessened. Yes, this is a new state of mind she has never experienced before.

Now she could tell her story for the first time. She had never told anyone before. She couldn't, she says. She didn't want to burden the children with it. It wasn't until they asked and the son became interested and obtained films and started digging deeper that she told them, as well as she could. That was after the first dose of the homeopathic remedy.

Grete shows her favorite photo - it is her son on a Baltic beach. "That's where I played - that's the Vistula Lagoon. At least my son could go and stand there - he went there for the wedding of the Russian too." Grete's son was a rail enthusiast and he took a steam train along the old route from Berlin to Königsberg. Greta herself did not want to come - she wouldn't have coped with that, but she asked her son to bring her some soil from her old home in East Prussia. After many setbacks, a Russian soldier helped him to carry out his task, which was against all the rules. Not long after, Sergej the Russian was standing at Grete's door. They communicated in English. "Sergej, how nice, what a lovely person. And then it became clear to me: You do not have the right to say 'Heimat' or homeland. Every person has the right to live where he was born. It was like that with him. He was born there and my boy was born here." Sometimes she remembers what her mother once said to her when she asked what Heimat was: "Well, it's here," she answered, "and when you have the first graves, then that's when you've put down roots." The graves of Grete's parents are nearby, and for the last five years, Alfred's too.

When he died, Grete wasn't with him. She had to be told. Alfred was at the neighbors' and had a heart attack. He just said, "I've got to go." Grete didn't scream or rage or cry. She just sat there as if she'd been shot. But her stomach didn't play up. That would have been unthinkable before. The shock came eight weeks later with high blood pressure, the inability to sleep, sweats, difficulty breathing and again, the inner agitation. Alfred had given her security and after his death she became quite dependent and couldn't cope well on her own.

Again, it is her daughter who sends Grete to Dr. Welte. In the meantime *Scorzerona* has appeared on the market, also in higher potencies. Grete is given five granules of Salsify potentised to 1M and soon after has a dream to do with her old theme: She is a young girl locked out of her house. She knows the right house number but can't get in because the number is wrong after all. For the first time in many years she wakes from the nightmare bathed in sweat. It is like a catharsis. After only a week she says that she has suddenly learned to be herself. Alfred is now with her. Now she can live with him and ask him for advice without going to the cemetery. He's always there. She keeps quiet about it - the others, "her own", would make fun of her. In the evenings when she sits down to rest, she apologizes to him sometimes saying, "Do you know, I haven't had any time for you today."

Grete's stomach problems have not recurred and neither have the fears or the nightmares. Sometimes she dreams of Alfred. It is a good dream. He goes on ahead and doesn't check the ice and she follows him confidently. The ice is safe. No cracking, no screams and no one sinks. Grete crosses the ice. She has firm ground under her feet. Grete has put down roots.

Commentary

Grete found her remedy herself. She couldn't get enough of it. But it wasn't until the salsify had lain in alcohol and the extract had been subjected to the mysterious homeopathic potentization process that the healing potential of the plant could work on the whole person. With her striking affinity to salsify, Grete led the homeopathic practitioner to a remedy that until then had not been revealed to homeopathy.

It is not that uncommon for people to have a special relationship with the substance that can heal them homeopathically. For example, two out of three patients who react well to the homeopathic remedy *Chocolate* (potentised chocolate) will have a craving for that particular sweet. Even though no homeopath would prescribe *Chocolate* based solely on this desire, the desire would make the homeopath think of the remedy and study its similarity to the patient. Patients whose remedy is a snake poison often have an extreme fear of snakes - even in pictures. Conversely, they may be fascinated by them. People taking part in homeopathic provings also often develop a special relationship to the original substance after taking the remedy, be it in their desires and aversions, in their fears or in their dreams. But in the case of *Scorzonera*, no proving had yet been conducted.

We know salsify as "poor man's asparagus", a vegetable that enriches the diet in Central Europe, especially in the winter months. This "winter asparagus" is rich in Inulin, a sugar which is fructose-rich and therefore suitable for diabetics. Inulin, not to be confused with the hormone Insulin, feeds the body's own intestinal bacteria and thus supports normal bowel function. In the Middle Ages wild salsify was used as a medicinal plant for the stomach and the gut. It was not grown as a vegetable until around 1700 and then as time went by, the healing properties of *Scorzerona hispanica* were forgotten. Salsify does not appear in the big encyclopedias of herbal medicine of today. Grete unearthed salsify as a medicinal plant in all senses of the word.

Using this remedy Grete's homeopath could, however, draw on experience of plants from the same botanical family. *Scorzerona* belongs to the Asteraceae or Compositae (composite) family. This is one of the largest plant families to which plants as disparate as lettuce, the carline thistle, and the daisy belong. Amongst the plants in this family already known to homeopathy, wild lettuce (*Lactuca virosa*) and chicory (*Cichorium intybus*) are the most closely related to salsify. In the case histories of patients who have been successfully treated with these homeopathic remedies, there are repeatedly situations in which these people were violently ripped out of their familiar environment and thrust into life-threatening conditions, similar to the situation that triggered Grete's history of suffering. Dr. Ulrich Welte therefore views being uprooted as a keynote for prescribing a remedy from this sub-family of the Compositae family.

Because of the unusual way in which Dr. Welte found the remedy for Grete, the description of the reasoning behind its choice has been kept to the end of the book. Such experiments should only be attempted when one has a good understanding of homeopathy and much experience in Classical prescribing. However, this particular story highlights succinctly what our method of treatment involves and what sets it apart from conventional medicine. As we have emphasized over and again, the distinguishing feature of homeopathy - apart from the Law of Similars - is the principle of strict individualization. Dr. Welte took this principle to the highest degree and produced a personal remedy especially for Grete - a remedy hitherto unknown. Dr. Welte was not guided by reflection or theoretical ideas - he followed the recommendation of an authority that knows Grete inside out. Grete's inner doctor had clearly told him what did her good and which remedy she needed. Dr. Welte concentrated on this one signal, potentised it and translated it into the language of homeopathy.

This brought to an end over fifty years of deep, inner suffering. And thus we come full circle to the story of Eloise who, thirty years after serious burns and a traumatic childhood, discovered the world anew and found her way back to life with the help of her individual remedy. Not every patient will experience such a dramatic transformation through homeopathy. But cases such as these, where someone really becomes whole again, stand over and over as shining examples of just what is possible with this amazing medical art.

Glossary

Aggravation In about a third of all homeopathic treatments, the patients' symptoms intensify for a short time before they get better. The remedy intensifies the symptoms which are already presenting and thus triggers the body's healing counter-reaction. For this reason, an aggravation within the disease picture is a good sign for the homeopath. But be aware that not every deterioration in the well-being of a patient after taking a homeopathic remedy is to be taken as a positive signal. New symptoms are by definition not the result of an aggravation but a sign that the patient is inadvertently proving the remedy. Therefore the homeopath should always be contacted if a remedy reaction is particularly strong or unusual.

Case Analysis In Hahnemann's words, once the homeopath has taken the case and documented the symptoms "the most difficult work is done." The next step is to compare the disease picture with the proving symptoms of various remedies. In order to do that, the patient's symptoms must be weighted and the wheat separated from the chaff. Of chief interest, according to the famous section 153 of Hahnemann's *Organon of Medicine,* are: "the more striking, singular, uncommon and peculiar (characteristic) signs and symptoms of the case of disease." With the help of a repertory, the homeopath finds the remedies which can cause exactly these symptoms. In order to choose the optimal simillimum, the homeopath studies the remedies in the Materia Medica and compares them with the disease picture. As well as this classical method of case analysis, several other methods have become established over the last few decades, above all the work with remedy families and other remedy classification systems. With the help of group analysis, as explained more fully in the commentary on chapter 8, lesser known or not fully proved remedies can be included in the choice of a homeopathic remedy.

Case Taking The method of taking the case history in homeopathy is very different to that of conventional medicine. Whilst conventional medicine is concerned with symptoms and objective findings which lead to a diagnosis, the homeopath is principally interested in the subjective condition, in individual signs of disease and personality traits. The homeopath asks what kind of person the patient is, what has made him ill, how he experiences his condition and how he reacts to his affliction. The aim of homeopathic case taking is to understand the patient with all his idiosyncrasies, to identify his personal and particular suffering at the current time, but also to view it in the context of his life story. Hahnemann wrote in section 83 of his work *Organon of Medicine*: "This individualizing examination of a case of disease … demands of the physician *nothing but freedom from prejudice and sound senses*, attention in observing and fidelity in tracing the picture of the disease." An important pre-condition he did not mention was that both homeopath and patient must be prepared to invest quite some time in the taking of a detailed biographical case.

Constitution This term usually refers to build, character or the classic temperaments. In this book it is used as described in the following quote by the eminent homeopath and psychoanalyst Edward C. Whitmont: "By constitution we mean the inherent tendency to react automatically according to fixed individual and characteristic patterns. Differences in constitutions become apparent through differing reactions to identical situations." Inherited and acquired aspects of the constitution provide the framework for health, growth and development and also for disease and stagnation on all levels. The constitution makes a person susceptible to particular types of stress and similarly to the type and location of particular diseases. A homeopathic remedy which reflects a person's readiness to react, his individual weak points and susceptibility is called his constitutional remedy. Whitmont writes: "It is only by seeking a therapeutic method that accepts the given pattern of reaction instead of disregarding it and working against it that we can avoid the patterns harming us. Only then are we able to successfully transform susceptibilities into potential strengths."

Diagnosis Like any doctor, homeopaths will always try to recognise a particular disease picture in a patient's complaints because this provides important information concerning the prognosis and thus whether treatment with homeopathy alone is suitable. However, the medical diagnosis of a disease is only of slight importance when choosing the simillimum. The homeopath tries to match the patient's symptoms to a particular remedy according to the Law of Similars. This remedy-based diagnosis is the basis for homeopathic treatment.

Dosage Dosage includes the choice of potency and the decision as to how many drops, granules or tablets should be taken and how often. As a rule of thumb, high potencies are given at longer intervals, often several weeks, whilst lower potencies up to 12X or 12 C and also the LM potencies are given more often, sometimes even several times a day. However, the dosage should always be tailored to the individual reaction of the patient.

Globules In some parts of the world these little spherical pellets or pillules are almost a trademark of homeopathy. Remedies can also be given in liquid form (in drops or spoonfuls), as tablets of various types, as powders or even in ampoules for injection. For remedies in solid form, sugar acts as the carrier onto which the potentized active ingredient, dissolved in a mixture of water and alcohol, is sprayed.

High Potencies The widespread scepticism relating to homeopathy mainly focuses on the issue of high potencies. A high potency means one greater than 23X, which has a dilution of 1 to 10^{23} (that is a ten with twenty three zeros). According to the calculations of the Austrian physicist Johann Josef Loschmidt, homeopathic remedies above the potency of 23X or C 12 contain no molecules of the original substance. The effect of the higher potencies can therefore not be directly due to the original substance as there are no molecules left. It is assumed that during and due to the process of succussion (vigorous shaking), information from the original substance is transferred to the solvent, for example through changes in its physical structure or its electromagnetic field. Even if the exact principles by which higher potencies work remain a scientific riddle, their effectiveness is proven time and again in clinical practice and clinical studies.

Law of Similars *Similia similibus curentur* - like cures like. In a few words this phrase sums up the core of homeopathy. It describes a natural law which was formalized by the German doctor Samuel Hahnemann over two hundred years ago. The name that he gave his new method comes from the Greek words *homoios*- same and *pathos* - suffering and it refers directly to this basic law of cure. A substance works homeopathically when it can produce the same complaint in a healthy person that it cures in a sick patient. A remedy must be able to cause an artificial disease which corresponds to the major characteristics of the condition of the patient.

Materia Medica A reference work in which homeopathic remedies and their symptoms are listed is called a Materia Medica. Some of these encyclopedias solely contain symptoms from provings and poisonings and others are expanded to include findings from clinical practice and clinical observations of cured patients. Today, the complete Materia Medica with its thousands of remedies, the treasure-trove of homeopathic experience collected over the last two centuries, is available as specialist computer software. The search functions of these programs simplify the task of comparing symptoms and remedies enormously.

Potency Whilst searching for the optimal dose, Dr. Hahnemann experimented with very small amounts of substances. He made the surprising discovery that when subjected to a particular mechanical process, the remedies in minute doses worked better than the undiluted source material. On the strength of this observation, he developed a special production process for homeopathic remedies that he called potentization. The source material is diluted and succussed in stages. The substance is diluted with a mixture of water and alcohol or with lactose and is dynamised either by vigorously shaking (succussing) liquid solutions or grinding a substance with lactose in a mortar. The level of dilution is shown as an Arabic numeral followed by the ratio in which the substance is diluted from substance to carrier, indicated by a Roman numeral. A remedy of potency 12 C will have been diluted and succussed twelve times in the ratio 1:100. 'X' stands for the ratio 1:10 and the LM or Q potencies are diluted by 1:50,000 at every stage of dilution.

Provings Homeopathic remedies are tested on healthy people in order to determine which complaints and unhealthy conditions can be caused by a remedy and thus, according to the Law of Similars, can also be cured by it. Participants in such an experiment (or proving), mostly homeopaths themselves, take a potentized substance and note every change in the way they feel and every symptom that they observe in themselves. Even though some provers may experience subjectively considerable complaints, the organism is not harmed by taking the potentized remedy. These are temporary functional disturbances that tail off after a few days if the remedy is not repeated. The voluntary testers usually do not know which remedy they are proving or whether they are taking the remedy or a placebo (a dummy medicine without the active ingredient). These precautions help to identify the symptoms which definitely come from the remedy. After a number of weeks, the notes from all the provers are reviewed and a first draft of the remedy picture is made from the symptoms collected.

Remedy Picture The picture that a homeopath forms of a patient from taking his case is compared to a remedy picture using the Law of Similars. When doing this, the particulars of a remedy, the unusual characteristics which distinguish it from other remedies, are to be understood in the same way that the individuality of the patient is. In the remedy picture, the many symptoms from the proving of the substance, from knowledge of the effect of toxic dosages and from documented curative effects from its use fit together like the pieces of a puzzle to form a picture which the experienced homeopath can recognise in his patient.

However, it is in the nature of similarity that the symptoms presented by a patient can reflect the pictures of more than one remedy, so it is sometimes not easy for the homeopath to choose the simillimum from a group of similar remedies or similes.

Repertory A repertory is a reference work that is constructed the opposite way around to a Materia Medica; in other words it is organised according to symptoms rather than remedies. Under each particular symptom or rubric in the repertory, the homeopath finds listed all the remedies that have caused this symptom either in a proving or in a poisoning, and the remedies which have been particularly useful in treating this symptom. Repertories are now available as computer software as well as the Materia Medica. When you look up a patient's main signs of disease and complaints with the help of such a computerised encyclopedia of symptoms and collect the relevant rubrics, you get a 'hit list' of homeopathic remedies common to all or most of the rubrics. Then the homeopath can check for each remedy to what extent the remedy and disease picture coincide. Despite all the electronic refinements available, the evaluation of a repertorisation still requires much experience.

Simile and Simillimum The simile is a successful remedy chosen according to the Law of Similars. Because similarity is not a precise term and cannot be exactly defined, there can be several remedies similar to a particular disease picture. The remedy that reflects the patient's condition best and works deepest is sometimes called his simillimum and sometimes called his constitutional remedy. (See **Constitution**.)

Periodic Table of the Elements
Modified according to Jan Scholten

Stage	1	2	3	4	5	6	7	8	9	10	11	12	13	14	15	16	17	18
Series 1	H																	He
Series 2	Li	**Be**	B							C					N	O	F	Ne
Series 3	**Na**	Mg	Al							Si					P	S	Cl	Ar
Series 4	K	Ca	Sc	Ti	V	Cr	Mn	Fe	Co	Ni	Cu	Zn	Ga	Ge	**As**	Se	Br	Kr
Series 5	Rb	Sr	Y	Zr	Nb	Mo	Tc	Ru	Rh	Pd	Ag	Cd	In	Sn	Sb	Te	I	Xe
Series 6	Cs	Ba	La	Hf	Ta	W	Re	Os	Ir	Pt	Au	Hg	Tl	**Pb**	Bi	Po	At	Rn
Lanthanides				Ce	Pr	**Nd**	Pm	Sm	Eu	Gd	Tb	Dy	Ho	Er	Tm	Yb	Lu	

Be = Beryllium
Nd = Neodymium
Pb = Plumbum/lead
Na = Natrium/sodium
As = Arsenicum/arsenic

Bibliography

1. A Stranger in Her Own Skin – *Carbo animalis*

Hahnemann, Samuel. The Chronic Diseases: Their Peculiar Nature and Their Homoeopathic Cure [1828]. Translated from the German by L. H. Tafel. 1896. Reprint, New Delhi: B. Jain Publishers, 2003.

Vithoulkas, George. The Science of Homeopathy. New York: Grove Press, 1980.

Vithoulkas, George. Materia Medica Viva. Volume 7. London: Homeopathic Book Publishers, 1997.

2. Blessed Art Thou, Maria – *Cicuta virosa*

Hahnemann, Samuel. *Materia Medica Pura* [1811]. Translated from the German by R. E. Dudgeon. 1880. Reprint in 2 vols., New Delhi: B. Jain Publishers, 2003.

Kent, James Tyler. *Lectures on Materia Medica*. 1905. Reprint, New Delhi: B. Jain Publishers, 1999.

Kent, James Tyler. *Repertory of the Homoeopathic Materia Medica*. [1897]. Revised edition as Kent's Final General Repertory of the Homoeopathic Materia Medica, revised by P. Schmidt & D. Chand [1974]. Reprint, New Delhi: National Homoeopathic Pharmacy, 1980.

Schroyens, Frederik. *Synthesis: Repertorium Homeopathicum Syntheticum*. Edition 9.1. London: Homeopathic Book Publishers, 2004.

Vithoulkas, George. *Materia Medica Viva*. Volume 8. London: Homeopathic Book Publishers, 1997.

3. The End of The Line – *Ignatia amara*

Coulter, Catherine. *Portraits of Homeopathic Medicines*. Vol 2. St Louis: Quality Medical Publishing, 1988.

Kent, James Tyler. *Lectures on Materia Medica*. 1905. Reprint, New Delhi: B. Jain Publishers, 1999.

4. Lovesick – *Cypraea eglantina*

Schadde, Anne. *Cypraea eglantina* in Schadde, Anne and Hansel, Jürgen. *Listening to Stone, Wood and Shell*. Mumbai: Homoeopathic Medical Publishers, 2004.

5. The Land Beyond the Desert - *Folliculinum*

Assilem, Melissa. "Folliculinum – Mist or Miasm?" *The Homœopath*, Vol. 11/1 (1991).

Martinez, Bruno. "Folliculinum – Efficacy in premenstrual syndrome." *British Homoeopathic Journal*, Vol. 79 (1990).

6. Red and Blue – *Conium maculatum*

Hahnemann, Samuel. *The Chronic Diseases: Their Peculiar Nature and Their Homoeopathic Cure* [1828]. Translated from the German by L. H. Tafel. 1896. Reprint, New Delhi: B. Jain Publishers, 2003.

Madaus, Gerhard. *Lehrbuch der biologischen Heilmittel.* Leipzig: Georg Thieme Publishers, 1935.

Clarke, John Henry. *A Dictionary of Practical Materia Medica*. 3 vols. 1900. Reprint, New Delhi: Indian Books & Periodicals Syndicate, undated.

Schroyens, Frederik. *Synthesis: Repertorium Homeopathicum Syntheticum.* Edition 9.1. London: Homeopathic Book Publishers, 2004.

Zandvoort, Roger van. *The Complete Repertory.* Leidschendam, Netherlands: Institute for Research in Homeopathic Information and Symptomatology, 2007.

7. The Lost Warrior – *Plumbum metallicum*

Sankaran, Rajan. *The Spirit of Homeopathy.* 3rd edition. Mumbai: Homoeopathic Medical Publishers, 2004.

Sankaran, Rajan: *The System of Homeopathy.* Mumbai: Homoeopathic Medical Publishers, 2001.

Scholten, Jan. *Homeopathy and the Elements.* Utrecht, Netherlands: Stichting Alonissos, 1996.

8. A Law Unto Himself – *Neodymium oxydatum*

Scholten, Jan. *Secret Lanthanides.* Utrecht, Netherlands: Stichting Alonissos, 2005.

9. Savita's Smile - *Beryllium metallicum*

Shah, Jayesh. *Into the Periodic Table: The Second Series.* Hamburg: Schröder und Burmeister Publishers, 2006.

10. A Part of the Family– *Colchicum autumnale*

Sankaran, Rajan. *The Soul of Remedies.* Mumbai: Homoeopathic Medical Publishers, 1997.

Sankaran, Rajan. *An Insight Into Plants.* Volume 1. Mumbai: Homoeopathic Medical Publishers, 2002.

11. The Poison of Fear – *Natrium arsenicosum*

Scholten, Jan. *Homeopathy and Minerals.* Utrecht, Netherlands: Stichting Alonissos, 1993.

12. The Prince in the Caul or The Child of Fortune - *Conchiolinum*

Allen, Timothy Field. *Encyclopedia of Pure Materia Medica.* 1887. Reprint, New Delhi: B.Jain Publishers, 1975.

Glossary

Hahnemann, Samuel. *Organon of Medicine.* 5th/6th Editions. [1833]. 5th Edition translated from the German by R. E. Dudgeon [1849] with amendments from 6th Edition manuscript by W. Boericke [1922]. Reprint, New Delhi: B. Jain Publishers, 1986.

Whitmont, Edward C. *Psyche und Substance: Essays on Homeopathy in the Light of Jungian Psychology.* 3rd revised edition. Berkeley, California: North Atlantic Books, 1992.

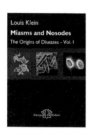

Louis Klein
Miasms and Nosodes
The Origins of Diseases - Volume I
hb, 400 pp, € 45.00

Louis Klein is a homeopathic pioneer who uses many previously unknown nosodes. He describes new miasms and defines the existing miasms anew in a demystified and easily understandable way. According to him, miasms are nothing more than resulting chronic states of infectious diseases, and nosodes are the remedies derived from these infectious diseases. On the basis of his broad clinical experience he attributed many known remedies to miasmatic states. A miasmatic state becomes the core idea around which similar remedies are grouped.

For example Tetanus miasm signifies states of spastic paralysis, which can be treated with remedies of this miasmatic realm. Apart from its prototype, the Tetanus nosode, Tetanus miasm incorporates remedies like Angustura, Hypericum, and Helodrilus. So this new miasmatic classification of remedies is highly practical and useful.

This book is the first of a series of 3 volumes, where Louis Klein describes the history of miasms and his systematic new approach to this concept of disease.

In his first volume, he presents the following categories:
- Burkholderiales and the Pertussis miasm
- Clostridiales and the Tetanus miasm
- Corynebacteriaceae and Diphtheria
- Mycobacterium and the Tubercular and Leprosy miasm including newly proven Johneinum (Crohn's disease)
- Parasitic Protozoa and Parasitic miasms such as the Malaria miasm and the Toxoplasmosis miasm
- Enterobacillales including the Bach Bowel Nosodes, the Typhoid miasm, the Yersinia miasm and similar remedies belonging to theses miasms.

Many of the miasms are demonstrated through several excellent cases, which speak for themselves.

This book is a class of its own. As Rajan Sankaran is known for plant remedies and Jan Scholten for the periodic table, Louis Klein will be known for miasms and nosodes.

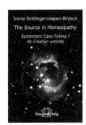

Irene Schlingensiepen-Brysch
The Source in Homeopathy

Systematic Case Taking I - As Creation unfolds

hb, 200 pp, € 39.00

The information about every patient's simillimum is already present in his or her subconscious mind. It can be revealed directly by the patient himself. A skilled homeopath can facilitate the patient's access to his own deep inner knowledge.

In years of meticulously documented case-taking, Irene Schlingensiepen has developed the basis of this groundbreaking, source-based approach. She describes how to accompany the patient's journey into his subconscious world and encourage him to express the specific source of his simillimum. A remedy, which might not even be known to the homeopath or currently found in any rubric. Such a source-based prescription will most likely produce amazingly deep healing results.

The method is illustrated by the essence and cases of 24 remedies derived from a cosmic origin, like Sol, Helium, Positronium, Volcano and its precious stones, Brass or Meteorite, many of which in themselves are almost unknown terrain. An exciting venture into pristine territory.

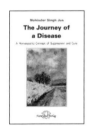

Mohinder Singh Jus
The Journey of a Disease

A Homeopathic Concept of Suppression and Cure

hb, 288 pp, € 29.00

Suppressive therapy can induce a shift of symptoms. Suppression can complicate chronic diseases and set them on a dangerous journey through the system. This odyssee is what the author describes as 'the journey of a disease'. He exposes many mainstream medical practices as suppressive therapy of symptoms. On the background of Hahnemann's theory of miasms, Mohinder Singh Jus paints vivid and detailed pictures of psoric, sycotic, syphilitic and tubercular forms of disease. Written in simple language, it has helped homeopaths and laypeople to understand classical homeopathy, which may cure chronic diseases and reverse suppression.

Many homeopaths recommend this book to their patients as part of the therapy, as they will understand the homeopathic principles and follow them on the journey to the right cure.

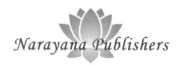

Narayana Publishers

Blumenplatz 2, 79400 Kandern, Germany
Tel: +49 7626-9749700, Fax: +49 7626-9749709
info@narayana-publishers.eu
Online Shop: www.narayana-publishers.eu

Our bookstore offers a wide range of English homeopathic titles and all German homeopathic books.

We deliver books to homeopathic schools and training courses at special conditions.

Ulrich Welte
Colors in Homeopathy
Wire-O, 82 pp, 120 colors with Color Repertory and a Manual, € 58.00

This is a unique color repertory. The color preference expresses the inner state of a patient directly, and as such it is a significant and specific homeopathic symptom. It has been helpful to indicate or confirm the correct diagnosis of a remedy in many cases. 18 years of clinical experience in thousands of cases stand behind this publication. Foreword by Jan Scholten.

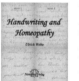

Ulrich Welte
Handwriting and Homeopathy
Hb, 344 ppp, 750 handwriting samples related to 315 remedies, € 28.00

Personality structure expresses itself in handwriting. Handwriting is a frozen image of motion patterns. So handwriting is a significant clinical background symptom of great depth. It is well worth learning to read this 'script inside the script'.

This book is a reference work to compare handwritings in homeopathic practice. Numerous case descriptions illustrate the usefulness of this new symptom and serve as a practical guide to its successful application.